The American Yoga Association's

New Yoga
Challenge

The American Yoga Association's

New Yoga Challenge

Powerful Workouts
for Flexibility, Strength,
Energy, and Inner Discovery

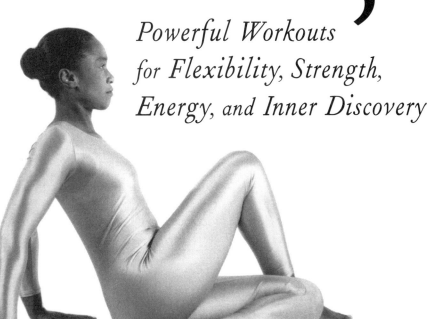

Alice Christensen, Founder, American Yoga Association

Produced by The Philip Lief Group

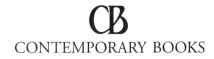

CONTEMPORARY BOOKS

Library of Congress Cataloging-in-Publication Data

Christensen, Allice.
   The American Yoga Association's new yoga challenge : powerful
workouts for strength, flexibility, and inner discovery / by Alice Christensen.
      p.   cm.
   Includes index.
   ISBN 0-8092-3175-1
   1. Yoga—Health aspects.   I. American Yoga Association.   II. Title.
RA781.7.C4864   1996
613.7'046—dc20   96-44651
                                                                      CIP

Reader's Note:
The techniques and suggestions presented in this book are not intended to substitute for proper medical advice. Consult your physician before beginning thls or any new exercise program. The author, the American Yoga Association, the producer, and the publisher assume no responbibility for injuries suffered while practicing these techniques. The American Yoga Association does not recommend this book for pregnant or nursing women or for children under 16 years of age. If you are elderly or have any chronic or recurring conditions such as high blood pressure, neck, or back pain, arthritis, heart disease, and so on, seek your physician's advice about which techniques you should avoid.

The models in this book are all students of the American Yoga Association: Patrick Benz, founder and president of an international plastics development company; Brenda Brown, police officer; Kent England, contractor; Artie Guerin, tennis instructor; Steve Honeyager, maintenance supervisor; Lea Jackson, interior designer; Nancy Leland, Yoga instructor; and David Tipton, attorney.

Cover design by Monica Baziuk
Interior design by Hespenheide Design
Exercise photos by Evelyn England, Sage Productions
Models' hair and makeup by Ashley Vann-Kingston
Drawings by Lea Jackson

Published by Contemporary Books
A division of NTC/Contemporary Publishing Group, Inc.
4255 West Touhy Avenue, Lincolnwood (Chicago), Illinois 60712-1975 U.S.A.
Copyright © 1997 by the American Yoga Association and the Philip Lief Group, Inc.
Printed in the United States of America
International Standard Book Number: 0-8092-3175-1

00 01 02 03 04 05 ML 19 19 18 17 16 15 14 13 12 11 10 9 8 7 6 5 4 3 2

This book is dedicated to my teachers:
Rama of Haridwar and Kashmir,
and Lakshmanjoo of Kashmir.

Contents

Acknowledgments

I would like to thank all the people who have helped with the preparation of this book, including: Pattie Cerar, Paige Christopher, Linda Gajevski, Corrine Goodman, Roger Hess, Cynthia Ingalls, Nancy Leland, and Patricia Rockwood.

Introduction

The American Yoga Association's New Yoga Challenge will appeal to those of you who enjoy any type of physical activity as well as those of you who have practiced Yoga before and wish to learn more. You don't have to be in perfect physical shape to enjoy this book, and you don't have to have any previous experience in Yoga. However, you will get the most out of this book if you are at least moderately active, because the approach here is more rigorous than in beginning-level Yoga manuals.

In Yoga, *challenge* is determined not only by the difficulty of the techniques you practice, but also by the attitudes with which you approach your practices and the increased awareness that may prompt you to scrutinize other aspects of your life. The chapter titles in this book suggest the qualities that these Yoga routines will help develop in you: attention, energy, strength, flexibility, focus, steadiness. As you work at learning these vigorous sequences, you will be challenged to stretch your horizons in other ways. The meditations, fantasy techniques, and discussion topics will suggest how to change your view of yourself and explore new possibilities for inner growth.

The teaching of Yoga in this country has become quite physically oriented since I first began teaching in the mid-1960s. Many people now see Yoga simply as an alternative form of physical exercise, but Yoga is a combination of techniques that must be done together. By practicing meditation and breathing techniques as well as the Yoga asan routines (*asan* means "posture"), you will enjoy a safe, comprehensive Yoga challenge that will bring shining health and a deep, enduring happiness within yourself.

Even if you are limited by some physical condition, you can be challenged by approaching Yoga practice with the idea of constantly increasing your awareness of yourself and your life. I have tried to present the material in this book so that it will be usable to anyone, regardless of physical condition or age. Some of the exercises are very difficult, but you always have a choice; you can start by practicing just part of a routine until you gain the strength and stamina to do the complete routine. Choose techniques that you like to do and that you can do without pain.

There is a parable told by Plato about a man who lived his entire life in a dark cave. One day he ventured out into the sunlight, and he was so frightened and overwhelmed that he ran back into the cave, determined never to try leaving his familiar surroundings again. Most of us are like this man, aware only of the limited resources of our mind and body that are apparent in our external lives. By accepting the challenge of Yoga, you are taking the courageous step of saying that you want to expand your knowledge about yourself, even if it

means confronting massive changes. This type of transformation, from the darkness of limitation and ignorance into the light of freedom and choice, is represented in myth by the serpent who guards the gates of knowledge. This serpent, of course, also represents the force of *kundalini*, the energy of consciousness that is released by the physical and mental techniques of Yoga (see "The Kundalini Experience" in Chapter 9). As kundalini begins to move, the experience joins your outer, seemingly conscious self to your inner, unknown self for an experience of completeness that dissolves feelings of separateness. The word *Yoga* comes from the Sanskrit *yug*, meaning to join or yoke; the ultimate experience in Yoga is this union of all parts of yourself to become a powerful, intensely strong person.

A Yoga student who desires to go beyond the simple "bending and breathing" of beginning practice is like the man in Plato's story who, instead of running back into the cave, decides to leave its familiar walls and venture into the outside world even though it seems so terrifying at first. The classic tale of the person who sets off on this type of heroic journey against massive odds is told all over the world—Theseus, Gawain, and the Buddha are just a few examples of the many legendary heroes. The hero's adventure is, of course, the way all cultures represent the journey that all of us attempt in one way or another—the journey to find out who we are and why we were born—in short, to find meaning in life.

The path can be a daunting one, and not everyone is able to follow it through to the end. The *Bhagavad Gita* (one of the classic texts on the philosophy and practice of Yoga) states that perhaps one in five hundred thousand people attempts to practice Yoga. Since you are interested enough in Yoga to read this book, you must be one of those extraordinary individuals, and I congratulate you on the heroic adventure you are beginning.

Challenge in Yoga means moving ever deeper in thought, gently testing your limitations, being ready and able to face change. By working your way through this book step by step, you will learn to challenge yourself physically and mentally at the speed most comfortable for you. Even when it is rigorous, Yoga should be enjoyable; if you approach it correctly, you will look forward to your daily practice as if you were on your way to a meeting with a good friend—a friend who turns out to be yourself. Your daily practice will then become a catalyst for expansion and self-discovery.

In order to maintain this mythological transformation, you need more than muscle power alone; you need the support of a healthy body, a balanced mind, and love—what I call a "grandmother experience." By this I mean that you need to develop the kind of love for yourself that supports you in a way similar to that time when you nestled into your grandmother's lap, supported and protected, while you were listening and learning as a child. When you are supported by love, you feel free to expand your mind and heart, try new ideas, and find the courage to change. The practice of Yoga provides support and courage to go beyond the seeming limitations in our lives.

The American Yoga Association's New Yoga Challenge begins with a brief outline of the necessary preparations for Yoga practice. If you have never practiced Yoga before, Chapter 1, "Foundation," will tell you what to wear, what kind of environment you need, and other essential information about how to make your Yoga practice most successful.

This chapter also includes some vital information about diet. Yoga renews energy and strength, but it requires the support of proper nutrition (as well as adequate rest and other stress-management principles) to do so. If your diet is deficient, you will not have the resources to carry out the rigorous routines presented in this book—let alone to sustain the mental and emotional changes of the hero's journey. If you are a great "starter" and a poor "finisher," it's very possible that a proper diet is the missing factor needed to carry you to the finish line.

Chapter 2, "Attention," teaches you the important techniques of warming up, breathing, and meditation, which you should always include in your daily practice. Several breathing techniques are presented, along with instructions about when and how to practice them. The meditation procedure is presented in both a lying down and a seated version; begin with the position that is most comfortable for you.

The third chapter, "Fantasy," introduces an important idea: that we are the result of our fantasy picture of ourselves. Most people don't realize that this fantasy can become rigid and block change. By using this book, you will find that you and your fantasy of yourself can grow and change together. I have discovered that unless your fantasy of yourself changes, you cannot bring about change in yourself. Fantasy allows you to reach for the impossible. My teacher Lakshmanjoo used to say that all real change begins in the mind, and in this chapter I will show you how to start that process in yourself with two easy and effective techniques. The "Hall of Space" is a

fantasy technique that allows the hidden, inner experience within you to emerge. It can be used as an immediate solution to whatever concerns or problems are drawing your mind away from silence in meditation. The "I Love You" Fantasy Technique increases self-confidence and improves self-image; this is the best technique for building the reservoir of love that is so necessary for a strong hero.

Chapters 4 through 8 present seven different types of challenging routines, each with a different focus. Chapter 4, "Energy," introduces one of the most important sequences, the Sun Salutation, as well as a routine specially designed to remove fatigue and increase energy. In Chapter 5, "Strength," you will learn a very strenuous routine to build strength and stamina and prevent the weak joints that often result from excessive—and inexpert— emphasis on limbering. Stretching is addressed in Chapter 6, "Flexibility," with a general limbering routine for the back, hips, and knees. This routine can be used very effectively by athletes or to complement weight training. "Focus" is the subject of Chapter 7, in which you learn two routines: a short sequence of movements with longer holds to build concentration, and a balance routine that builds poise and strengthens the nervous system. Chapter 8, "Steadiness," introduces a routine that releases emotional tension that lodges in the body in various places, primarily the stomach and back.

The final chapter in this book, "The Powerful Individual," will help you see that Yoga is something you do according to your own needs and capabilities, not as a competitive sport in which you are constantly comparing yourself to models in a book or other students in a class. We have designed some simple, nonscientific questionnaires to help you assess your particular behaviors, feelings, and lifestyle. Using the recommendations offered with each section, you will see which routines and techniques will be most effective in helping you become more aware, healthy, and balanced. Refer to this chapter often as you progress, because if you practice Yoga regularly, you will change, and the guidelines in this chapter can give you the tools you need to support yourself during this process. Making yourself vulnerable to the constant opportunity for change is the greatest challenge of all, because it takes tremendous courage.

Throughout this book, I have included brief discussions on some concepts in Yoga philosophy that complement the topics in each chapter. If you wish to learn more about Yoga philosophy and practice, a

selection of recommended books is provided in Appendix B.

I find that most people welcome transformation when they realize that it can be approached without pain or fear. If you look upon *challenge* as an exciting opportunity rather than as a hardship, you will experience Yoga as an electric, positive part of your life that you will never want to be without. I have been practicing Yoga for over 45 years now, and I must say that although the continual transformation is always challenging, it is never boring.

Although this book includes Yoga routines and concepts that are more challenging than beginning-level, one is, nevertheless, always a beginner in Yoga. The subject is so vast that we are dwarfed by its huge complexities. The really wonderful thing about it is that merely by doing a few exercises and a small amount of meditation and breathing each day, and by trying to behave ethically, the knowledge starts to come from within. Gradually you notice a greater capacity for work and sensitivity; a new, enjoyable flexibility; and great relief from stress. As your inner self and your outer self become one, it is as if another complete person has been added to yourself, making you extremely strong, and able to live life with great depth and competency. I wish you every success as you continue your hero's journey in Yoga.

MY TEACHERS

The constant support and love of my teachers has sustained me greatly over the years. There comes a time in Yoga when a teacher is necessary, and I am fortunate to have known three great Yoga masters. Yoga bloomed in my life after an unforgettable experience one night in 1952. I was awakened out of a sound sleep by an intense white light that came toward me and entered me. I lost consciousness, and the next morning awoke at my usual time. As I sat up, the word *Yoga* filled my mind. I had never heard the word before. During the next few months I began to have intense visionary experiences. A large Indian man—who I later learned was Sivananda of Rishikesh—would appear to me at odd times of the day. At first I would run from the room in fright, but soon I got used to him, and he began to teach me in earnest. After a while he told me how to write to him in India, and we continued my lessons by correspondence. Sivananda taught me the basic techniques of Yoga—exercises, breathing, and meditation—which I practiced faithfully every day.

When Sivananda died unexpectedly, just before I was to go to India to study with him in person, I was devastated. He was my only human link with this strange practice that had taken over my life; in the early 1950s, no one I knew had any experience with Yoga. I tried to stop practicing, thinking that I could not go on without him, but soon the inexorable push of Yoga took over and I began again.

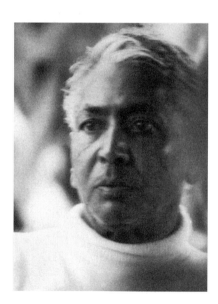

Rama of Haridwar and Kashmir

A few years later I received a call from an Indian research chemist who was living in the area. He told me that his guru was coming from India and asked if I would like to meet him. I rushed to the airport, and a small brown man in a Kashmiri bathrobe walked straight over to me and said, "Alice, I have come for you." This was Rama of Haridwar, who became my guru and guided me through nearly a decade of practice both in the United States and India. Under his auspices, the American Yoga Association (then known as the Light of Yoga Society) was formed in the late 1960s with a small group of students.

Rama died in 1972 in the United States. Before his death, he had told me that I should go to Kashmir to see a friend of his named Lakshmanjoo, who would continue my training. I went, as instructed, in 1974, and presented

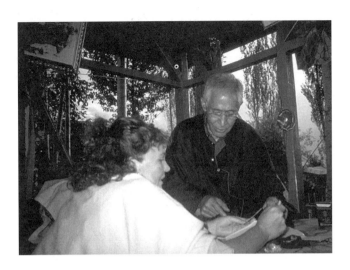

Alice in class with Lakshmanjoo in his teahouse in Kashmir

myself to this great master of Kashmir Shaivism. He accepted me as his student, and I still follow all the practices of a student to this day.

I know how difficult it is to find competent instruction in Yoga. This book contains information on the minimum qualifications I feel a teacher must have (see "How to Choose a Yoga Teacher" in Chapter 9). If you are lucky enough to find a competent teacher, your practice will be greatly enhanced. If you cannot find a teacher, you can use the instructions in this book as your teacher. I have written this book with this thought in mind—that the force of Yoga will shine through the sentences and illustrations so you will have exactly what you need to progress.

The American Yoga Association's

New Yoga
Challenge

1
Foundation

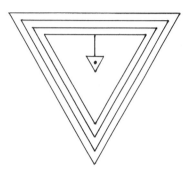

*The creative force of the universe and
its three qualities of nature*

How to Use This Book

This book has been designed to show you how to use Yoga techniques for a vigorous physical workout and guide you in using Yoga meditation and other inward-directed practices. Even if you've practiced Yoga before, I strongly recommend that you thoroughly familiarize yourself with the information in the first two chapters before beginning to practice the more vigorous routines. This chapter, Chapter 1, explains how to get started in Yoga in terms of equipment, scheduling, and so forth. Chapter 2 gives you complete instructions for (1) an essential warm-up routine, (2) the various breathing techniques that are recommended throughout the various routines, and (3) relaxation and meditation.

The special binding of this book allows you to lay the book flat on the floor in front of you as you practice. Always read through the instructions several times before trying an exercise so you won't have to interrupt the sequence to consult the book.

Be sure to check with your physician before beginning this or any new exercise program, especially if you have any chronic health conditions such as high blood pressure, arthritis, back or neck problems, or heart disease. Some of the more difficult exercises include variations for those with physical limitations, but only you and your physician can decide what's best for you to do. Never push or strain to the point of pain or exhaustion, and take frequent rest breaks.

CLOTHING, EQUIPMENT, AND ENVIRONMENT

There is no need to buy special exercise clothing; just wear clothes that are loose, warm, and comfortable—or stretchy, like leotards. Try to use your Yoga clothes only for Yoga. Avoid belts or other constricting garments. Practice the exercise portion of your routine in bare feet, but put on socks before you get settled for breathing and meditation. Have a sweater, shawl, or sweatshirt handy and put it on for meditation—even if you don't feel cold. Your body temperature will drop during meditation and you should not allow yourself to become chilled.

Choose a large towel, a small blanket, or a mat to do your exercises on even if your room is carpeted; this will help create an atmosphere conducive to daily practice. If the mat is not large enough for your entire body to fit on it, be sure your head is on the mat when you are lying down. Try to use this mat only for Yoga. Choose one or two firm cushions to sit on for breathing exercises, and use them only for Yoga also.

It's best to practice in a quiet, private space with a door that can be closed. The temperature of the room should be comfortable—neither too warm nor too cold. It helps to practice in the same room every day, at the same time; you're more likely to enjoy daily practice if it becomes habitual. This also allows your Yoga session to take less effort, freeing your mind for new experiences.

SCHEDULING

If you live with others, ask them to give you some uninterrupted time every day for Yoga. If you have never practiced Yoga before, start with a daily total practice time of twenty to thirty minutes (including breathing and meditation as well as exercise). As you progress, you'll probably naturally increase that time to about forty-five minutes or even more, depending on your desire. Some of the routines in this book may take longer—but remember, you don't always have to do the entire routine to benefit from Yoga.

The time of day that you practice is less important than practicing every day. Choose the time of day that is best for your schedule and lifestyle. Yoga can be a valuable help if it is practiced as part of your reentry routine—for instance, during the hour or so when you are winding down from work and turning your attention to your home life. By using Yoga as a transition between the outside world and the world of home and family, you can create a happier space wherever you are. Whatever time of day you choose to practice Yoga, you will find that the feelings of centeredness and well-being that Yoga brings you will be a valuable addition to any relationship—even if you live alone. You will find your creativity blooming without effort when you give yourself this private time every day.

An ideal Yoga routine consists of exercise, breathing, meditation, and fantasy techniques. The techniques complement each other when done consecutively. If you have small children or an extremely hectic lifestyle, however, you may not be able to negotiate as much time as you need all at one time. In that case, it's fine to split up your practice and do the various techniques at different times during the day. You can even do some techniques at work at your desk or in the bathroom. Try taking a "meditation break" instead of a coffee break in the middle of the day and see how easily the rest of your day goes. Find a private place away from the telephone, or sit in your parked car.

No matter how much time you are able to set aside each day for

Yoga practice, the important point is to practice *something* every day. You will not progress in Yoga unless you practice it once in every twenty-four-hour period. Yoga operates on many levels, and it takes time to become aware of the more subtle effects, but the cumulative effect of placing your mind and body in the positions of Yoga every day will show immediate results. You will see a marked difference after only about a week of daily practice.

Try to schedule your Yoga session at least two hours after a heavy meal or caffeinated beverages. Never practice Yoga under the influence of alcohol. So-called recreational drugs and Yoga definitely do not mix. If you use drugs—even occasionally—you risk great damage to yourself, both physically and mentally. The intensive physical and mental exercises outlined in this book demand great care for yourself as a student.

WOMEN'S ISSUES

Menstruation. Yoga has a strong effect on the hormonal system that will help relieve symptoms of PMS and generally keep you healthier and stronger. Because of the changes in body chemistry during the menstrual period, you should not practice Yoga asans during the days of heaviest bleeding. You may do a few simple stretching warm-ups, but avoid anything that compresses the abdominal area either forward (such as the Sun

Poses) or backward (such as the Cobra), or inverted poses (such as the Shoulder Stand). Fill in your regular practice time with a longer relaxation and more rest on those days.

Pregnancy. I recommend that you not practice Yoga asans during the first trimester when your body is still adjusting to its new function. After that time, with your doctor's permission, you can practice the modified routines that are described in two of my previous books, *The American Yoga Association Beginner's Manual* and *20-Minute Yoga Workouts* (see Appendix C).

Nursing. Because of the hormonal changes that occur during nursing and possible effects on the child, I recommend that you not practice Yoga asans until you have completely weaned your baby. It is very beneficial for you to continue with breathing and meditation, however, and you can stay active with other exercise programs.

Attitudes

Many people who approach Yoga for the challenge of a vigorous workout believe that they are not practicing correctly if they are not working up a sweat. Although many of the sequences in this book are quite rigorous, it is important to pay attention to such factors as making a smooth transition between positions, making sure that your body is positioned cor-

rectly, breathing properly, and keeping your mind focused and quiet.

More important than pushing your body to perspire is understanding the Asan Point, the culminating point of each asan. This is an important part of each exercise, and you will find that doing it correctly is quite challenging. During the Asan Point, for a moment or two your body is motionless, your breath is held, and you try to stop thinking. You may be surprised at how hard it is to sustain this throughout an entire asan sequence!

When you are practicing the Asan Point correctly, you will experience a double benefit from Yoga, because you are uniting a physical position with a mental position. This is one way Yoga differs from most calisthenics or casual sports, where it usually doesn't matter how you position your mind while you are exercising. In Yoga, mastery of the physical positions is only part of the goal—and even then, *mastery* does not mean attaining the extreme flexibility and strength to perform the asans to match the pictures in a book; it means simply doing the exercise to the very best of your ability and with your full concentration *at the present time, in your present physical condition.* I hope you can see now how ludicrous it would be to try to compare yourself to anyone else when you are practicing Yoga correctly. The competitive atmosphere of a gym is inappropriate in Yoga.

Those who believe that Yoga should be strenuous often equate success with suffering. Many people force themselves into Yoga positions, causing great pain and sometimes injury. I have always believed that Yoga should be enjoyed, not endured as a type of penance. Why should you force yourself to do something that is painful? To me, that would be harming yourself, contradicting one of the most important ethical guidelines in Yoga: nonviolence. The stereotypical picture of a Yogi (a serious practitioner of Yoga) is the emaciated *sadhu* (monk) lying on a bed of nails or suffering various other uncomfortable practices. This has nothing to do with Yoga. I've always believed that people who torture themselves this way must have a misplaced idea of bartering with God, so to speak—the age-old rationalization that suffering in this world is worthwhile because one will be rewarded in the next. Individual growth does not result from placing demands on the divine.

In Yoga philosophy, it is believed that one can attain the ultimate state of union with the self only while inhabiting a human body; therefore, practitioners are cautioned to take care of their bodies so as to keep them healthy and strong. In fact, Yoga asans were originally practiced not as an end in themselves but as a way to bring the body to optimum functioning and maintain it in that condition so that the mind can be free from distractions in meditation. This is still the intention for serious practitioners.

The connection between a strong, healthy body and a bright, alert mind is clear. When you are ill or fatigued, it is hard to think creatively, let alone still the mind for meditation. When you are rested and well, you can forget about your body for a few minutes at a time, which allows you to approach meditation without distracting thought. Yoga will help you remain well because, if practiced correctly, it will act to boost your immune system. The word *Yoga* comes from the Sanskrit *yug*, meaning to yoke or join, and this means a joining together of all parts of yourself. In order to practice Yoga correctly, you need a carefully balanced approach. Take every precaution to help yourself stay well: get enough rest, learn stress management techniques, eat a balanced diet, and exercise regularly (in addition to Yoga).

If you do get sick, you probably won't feel like practicing Yoga asans, and it's best not to do anything vigorous until you feel better. If you wish, you can do a few warm-ups and some simple stretches—there are even some exercises you can do in bed or in a chair—and you can always do a few minutes of breathing and meditation. It is more important to do a small amount of practice every day than it is to do a lot some days and nothing other days.

THE ASAN POINT

Posture becomes perfect when the effort to attain it disappears.

(Patanjali's Yoga Sutras)

In order to practice the routines in this book correctly, you should apply the concept of the Asan Point during the performance of all Yoga asans. The Asan Point teaches you to turn your attention inward; to increase the mental effect of the exercises. Once you have learned the physical mechanics of the asans, you might find your body moving through them automatically while your mind wanders off to other concerns, such as your shopping list, the menu for dinner, troubles with your boss, or what your kids are doing. You will still experience some benefits from doing the exercises, but the physical effects of Yoga asans are only a small part of the potential benefits; it is said that asans are 90 percent mental and only 10 percent physical. This mental effect is one of the most important ways in which you can attain a deeper experience of Yoga. Those who practice Yoga asans with the Asan Point are most likely to continue with Yoga because of the bridge that is formed between the mental and physical consciousness. Yoga asans practiced this way never become boring. They are no longer simply body movements; they produce creative intuition that shines forth from you like an unexpected treasure.

You practice the Asan Point at the culminating point of each asan. (These points are noted in the instructions for each exercise throughout this book by the words *Asan Point*.) Prepare for the Asan Point by following through with these three steps:

1. Be sure you are performing the holding position comfortably. Try to have correct alignment of the spine, placement of hands and feet, and weight distribution. This comfortable point will be different for every person according to his or her physical capabilities. A competitive attitude is counterproductive. After you've learned the asans, it's still a good idea to refer back to the book every few weeks to be sure you haven't forgotten any of the details. Make sure that you follow the instructions for each exercise exactly.

2. In every exercise, as you move toward the Asan Point, the breath is extremely important. Always breathe through your nose. If one or the other side of the nose is blocked, see "Alternate Nostril Breath" in Chapter 2 for suggestions on how to clear it. The sound of the breath should be audible and you should feel the breath becoming a steamlike sound in the back of your throat (see "Five Points for Effective Breathing" in Chapter 2 for more information about the sound of the breath). When you reach

your holding position, your breath will be held either in or out, depending on which exercise you are doing: (a) Interior hold: you've inhaled completely through your nose and are holding the breath in as you maintain the position briefly (as in the Cobra Pose); (b) Exterior hold: you've exhaled completely and are holding the breath out comfortably as you maintain the position (as in the Seated Sun Pose). Never hold your breath longer than you can comfortably. Remember, try not to strain.

3. Focus your eyes on one spot—generally at eye level, unless otherwise indicated (as in the Spine Twist). If you wish, you may use one of the diagrams that are at the beginning of each chapter in this book. You will notice that each diagram has a small black dot in the center. This dot represents the *bindu*, or the source of your concentration. Stare at the dot in the center of the diagram and try to think nothing.

Now you are ready to practice the Asan Point. With your body still and correctly positioned, your breath held in or out, and your gaze focused, try to stop all thought for that moment. This is the completion of the Asan Point. The silence in that point is extremely productive. Even a few moments of this practice can bring forth the brilliant, intuitive thought that leads into deeper practice in Yoga. Like baking a cake, you are mixing together all the right ingredients and placing the cake in the proper position; your efforts are transformed into a sweet result.

Do not attempt to hold the Asan Point too long; when you notice that you are becoming uncomfortable, come out of the position. After completing any pose, take a moment to stand or sit quietly and observe yourself. Then move on to the next position.

The Importance of a Good Diet

I began practicing Yoga in the early 1950s when hardly anybody knew about Yoga. By the time the American Yoga Association was formed, in the late 1960s, the United States was in turmoil with student uprisings, Vietnam War protests, and other causes, and many people were turning to Yoga and other Eastern practices for answers to the painful stress that we all were experiencing. Many of the young people who came to me to learn about Yoga during that time were quite unhealthy. Many had tried drugs or alcohol; many were malnourished; many were simply worn out by anxiety and the stress of a tumultuous lifestyle. In all cases, I found that before they could even begin to practice Yoga correctly they had to become healthy again, so I took great care that their first priority was to plan and execute a new diet. A good diet is the foundation of health. Without proper nutrition, your body will not be able to support the extra demands of an intensive Yoga practice—or, for that matter, any other important part of your life.

A proper diet complements the aspects of Yoga practice that naturally improve physical health. For instance, many Yoga asans help circulation by improving the elasticity of the blood vessels and pumping blood into the extremities. But if your diet is quite high in saturated fats, you may be contributing more to the congestion of your arteries than you are correcting. A diet that is moderate or low in fats helps keep your circulatory system healthy.

Similarly, Yoga practice helps you relax, both physically and mentally, by releasing muscle tension and improving respiration. But if your diet is high in caffeine, you are counteracting that effect by artificially stimulating your nervous and hormonal systems. A diet that is moderate in caffeine and other stimulants helps you maintain a relaxed, alert outlook.

You do not need to become a vegetarian to practice Yoga, although you will probably be healthier if you reduce your consumption of meat. Some advanced Yoga practices, however, can be dangerous if you are not a vegetarian. The chemical makeup of the body changes with a vegetarian diet, so the effect of these practices will be different. The Concentration Routine in Chapter 7 includes some "locks" (contractions of certain muscles along with a held breath) that, because of their intense effect on the subtle nervous system, should not be done unless you are a vegetarian. If you are not vegetarian, do the routine as

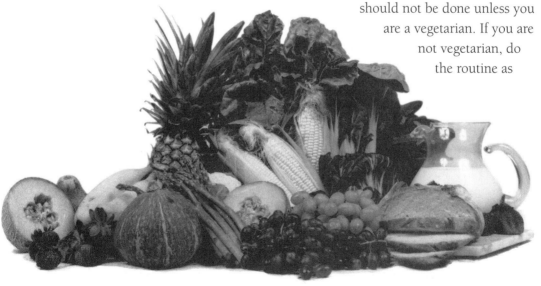

described, without the locks. Students who wish to begin the advanced practices of Mantric Yoga (the science of sound) must also be vegetarian, but few students decide to practice Yoga this seriously. I must add a comment about what I mean by *vegetarian*. Often I have met people who told me they were vegetarian because they didn't eat red meat, though they still ate fish and fowl. I do not consider this a vegetarian diet. To me, a vegetarian diet is not eating anything that looks back.

In their fervor to embrace everything associated with Yoga, some of my early students forced themselves to take on a vegetarian diet without really thinking, "Is this what I want to do?"; as a result, their vegetarian diet became a source of great hardship to them. I do not believe in forcing your body to change before it is ready; to me, that would be violent, and nonviolence is the first and foremost of the ethical guidelines required for serious Yoga practice. This means, above all, not harming yourself. So I would wait for meat to give you up instead of forcing yourself to give it up before your body is ready. In other words, let your body make the move. Educate yourself about nutrition and learn to become more aware of how food affects your body and mind. You will probably find that as you practice Yoga and your body becomes healthier, you naturally become more sensitive to what you eat, and this new awareness will help you make wise choices.

WHAT IS A GOOD DIET?

Opinions are constantly changing about what constitutes a good diet. In my opinion, food should be an appreciated resource, not an obsession that takes all of your time. I believe in eating a diet that is rich in natural foods, for instance, but I do not go out of my way to purchase organic produce exclusively. I believe that if your basic diet is healthy, a little "junk food" now and then will not hurt.

The current "food pyramid" (really a triangle) offered by the U.S. Department of Agriculture is a good general description of a healthy diet. In this schemata, the lower level of the triangle is made up of bread, cereal, rice, pasta, and baked goods. It is recommended that we eat six to eleven servings per day (a serving size is one-half bagel, one slice of bread, one-half cup of cereal, etc.). Whole grain breads and pastas and brown rice are healthier than white or bleached varieties, as are prepared cereals with the least amount of added sugar.

Next in the hierarchy are fruits, vegetables, and legumes. The recommendation is to eat four to six servings of vegetables and legumes and two to four servings of fruit per day. Eat a variety of fresh vegetables and fruit, as you like. If you can't use what you buy within a few days, buy fresh produce for the first part of the week and frozen for later use (fresh produce loses a great deal of its vitamin content if stored in your refrigerator for more than a few days). Buy fruit juices that are 100 percent fruit rather than those with added sweeteners.

On the next level we find dairy foods (two to three servings daily) and fish, poultry, meat, nuts, and eggs (one to two servings). Use low-fat or nonfat dairy products, and eat nuts and peanut butter sparingly. The calcium in dairy foods (and in other foods, of course) is essential for strong bones and to prevent or halt the development of osteoporosis in women approaching menopause. Most authorities recognize that it may be difficult for women to get adequate calcium from food, and therefore recommend calcium supplements. I have been advised that many calcium supplements do not dissolve completely in the system and therefore do not supply the calcium needed. I would suggest that you drink at least a quart of skim milk every day (this will also supply a great deal of your daily protein needs). Many of the challenging routines in this book include weight-bearing exercises that will help to increase bone density, but you should still support your practice with adequate dietary calcium. If you are a new vegetarian, count protein grams every day at first to be sure you are getting enough, and then check your intake every month or so. Adequate protein is very important for building muscle strength and for protecting against harmful stress reactions.

THE MYSTICAL MEANING OF MILK

The two great vessels, heaven and earth, have both been filled by the spotted cow with the milk of but one milking. Pious people, drinking of it, cannot diminish it. It becomes neither more nor less.

(*Taittiriya Upanishad*)

You may have noticed that in the section on diet I place great emphasis on drinking milk. The importance of adding milk to your diet goes a lot deeper than milk's physical properties of protein, calcium, and other nutrients. Milk has been called "the perfect food," and I believe that is an apt description, for more reasons than one.

Milk, in the most subtle sense, is the gift of life. Mythology is full of stories involving milk. India's tradition of revering cows comes from the story of the great divine cow called Kamadhenu, whose milk supports the life of the universe. In India, cows not only provide nourishment in the form of milk, their dung satisfies over half the fuel needs of the entire country and is also used as an antiseptic. In many agrarian societies, cows are considered the primary indication of wealth.

The god Vishnu, the preserver and protector of the universe, lies at rest on a huge coiled serpent, confidently asleep, supported by an ocean of milk. They float there happily, in a dream. This serpent is Kundalini, the great unseen energy in the spine that is awakened in Yoga practice. Even while they sleep, the ocean of milk is there to sustain them without any effort on their part.

In all beings, milk appears in the mother's body at the time of birth; this phenomenon is worshipped throughout the world. There are enchanting stories of the god Krishna who, in his baby years, was constantly dipping into his mother's butter pots to eat and play. My teacher Rama used to dip his thumbs in butter and massage the roof of my mouth and tongue. When I asked why he was doing this, he said, "It's a gift." Milk is never taken for granted in Yoga practice. It is always looked upon as the supreme gift that accompanies life.

When a Yoga student takes in any kind of good food, there are, ideally, two points of realization going on: one is that this food is physical nourishment to keep the body strong and healthy; the other is that worshipful thanks should be directed toward the primal source of the food. These two concepts are never separate in Yoga.

In Yoga you are asking your body to do extraordinary things and you want to give it the support it needs. Milk is one of the best foods to help you do this.

At the top of the triangle are sweets, fats, and condiments, to be eaten sparingly. Among oils, monounsaturates such as olive oil are the least harmful; new studies suggest that olive oil may actually help to raise levels of "good" cholesterol. Make your own salad dressings to avoid the extra sugar, salt, and fat in most commercial products. Using yogurt as a basis for salad dressings is a delicious and low-fat alternative.

In this top category I would add artificial or highly processed foods. Many additives, such as Nutrasweet and Olestra, are so new that we do not know what long-term effects they may have. We *do* know that artificial color and flavor, developed in the 1940s from coal tar, have been proven to be carcinogenic and also to cause hyperactivity in children. I suffered for a long time with an allergy to these additives and was eventually diagnosed by a wise allergist who told me that in order to break the cycle I had to refrain from all foods containing artificial colors and flavors for an entire year. It was quite difficult in those days, before product labeling was as strict as it is now, but I managed to find substitutes for the foods I was used to. I had to be alert to coloring in other products as well, such as toothpastes and mouthwashes.

WHAT DOES A YOGI EAT?

When I first started to practice Yoga, I eliminated onions and garlic from my diet very strictly after reading about it in books I found in the library. Later I realized that this was completely unnecessary and that those books had been written by people who wanted to become Hindus, not Yogis.

While I think it's important for Yoga students to pay attention to what they eat, I do believe that you should eat food that you like, that happily agrees with you, and that is fresh, wholesome, and attractive— food that will help support your body and mind. My teacher Rama told me that hot food feeds the bones of the body, and cold food feeds the nervous system; the best diet would include some of each.

If you decide you would like to become a vegetarian, take the time to count protein grams for a week or so until you become more familiar with the type of food you need to eat every day to get enough. The RDA for protein is only forty-five grams, but my own feeling is that the stress of modern life and the extra demands of Yoga practice require more. Eat plenty of low-fat or nonfat dairy foods, a moderate amount of unfertilized eggs or egg substitutes; whole grains, legumes, tofu and other soy products, and meat substitutes. The B vitamins are also extremely important for vegetarians; learn what they are and be sure you are getting plenty. A deficiency of B_{12} is a risk if you eliminate dairy products and eggs from your diet completely.

I never advise students to pursue austere diets. I have seen students become severely ill on extreme macrobiotic diets, for example, and I have never heard that Yoga requires fasting. Fasting seems to be more of a religious practice having to do with ideas about purification; this has nothing to do with Yoga. Many of the old books on Yoga offer advice about what and how to eat, but nowhere are Yoga students told to fast.

The *Hatha Yoga Pradipika* says, in fact, "The Yogi should not remain away from food more than three hours." The *Bhagavad Gita* advises moderation in food intake, and another source says, "The Yogi never completely fills his stomach." All advice points toward keeping the body healthy by feeding it regularly—but not overeating. I suggest that most food be taken at breakfast and lunch, and very little food at night, following the old saying, "Eat breakfast like a king, lunch like a prince, and supper like a pauper." The concept of "grazing" works, too, if you are disciplined enough to eat only a little at each of six small meals per day. In short, never stuff yourself, and never starve yourself.

If you have a problem with weight, I recommend trying to eat an entire head of lettuce every day plus a quart of skim milk, along with small quantities of whatever other foods you like. The calories in a quart of milk are about equal to one large muffin—and much more nutritious. The idea is that the lettuce and milk will fill you up so you will be less likely to snack on high-calorie foods.

Moderate behavior in all aspects of life is encouraged in Yoga. The nervous system becomes extremely sensitive in Yoga students, and what is needed is support and protection, not harsh austerities that weaken the system. Yoga is always about balance, never extremes.

Remember too that food not only feeds the physical body, it also affects the subtle systems of the body. A passage in the *Siva Samhita* reads as follows:

Of the four kinds of food (that which is chewed, that which is sucked, that which is licked, and that which is drunk), the life-giving fluid is converted into three parts. The best part (or the finest extract of food) goes to nourish the linga sharira *or subtle body (the seat of force). The second or middle part goes to nourish the gross body composed of seven humours. The third or most inferior part goes out of the body in the shape of excrement and urine. The first two essences of food are found in the* nadis *[the subtle pathways that carry energy throughout the body] and being carried by them, they nourish the body from head to foot.*

In Yoga, feeding the physical body is not the whole show! When you eat, you are feeding your inner self as well. You learn to worship food and its source as a gift given to you for support of life. This requires a thoughtful approach that does not allow a careless throwing of things down one's gullet.

My approach is to feed the nervous system foods that are supportive, wholesome, and calming. There are so many books about food now that are filled with warnings about various substances. I don't believe that it is possible—or wise—to strictly prescribe what someone should eat. Everyone has likes and dislikes; simply ask yourself, "Is this food agreeing with me? Is it helping me to be what I want to be?" In other words, as the saying goes, "you are what you eat." (Rama once observed a student eating a large helping of nuts and said, "If you want to be as big as a tree, eat nuts.")

Pay attention to what you are eating, notice the effect of food in your life, and enjoy it as a gift. Besides the restrictions of vegetarianism and my sensitivity to artificial substances, my own diet is varied and creative, and I delight in the wonderful variety that the world offers me.

2
Attention

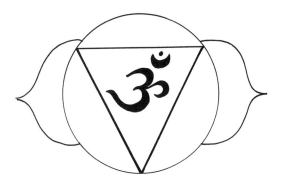

AUM: *A representation of the mind. Associated with the spot in the forehead between the eyebrows*

In this chapter you will learn some of the basic techniques that will help you become more aware of your body, breath, and mind. Beginning your routine with a series of light exercises to warm up gives you a chance to observe how your body is feeling so you can avoid injury. Warm-ups also help you begin the inner-directed process of quieting your mind. All the breathing techniques recommended for each routine are described here, including basic instructions in the *Complete Breath*—the foundation for all other breathing exercises—as well as more complex breathing techniques that affect respiration and awareness in various ways. You will also find complete instructions for relaxation and meditation in this chapter, including a special "quick relaxation" to use when you are pressed for time.

Warm-Ups

As you probably know, it's never a good idea to jump right into a vigorous workout without warming up; you risk injury or strain, and you won't gain as much awareness of your body as if you'd started more gradually. These simple warm-ups will help you get ready to exercise. They limber the large muscle groups, expand your breath, and gradually refine your attention—starting from the large movements of the body, moving on to the more subtle movement of the breath, and culminating in stillness of the mind.

Some days you may not feel like exercising at all, but Yoga must be practiced once every twenty-four hours to be effective, and the minimum number of daily exercises is three. If you start with these warm-ups—even saying to yourself that these will be the only exercises you do for the day—you will start to bring your mind into position for exercising. By the time the warm-ups are over, you may feel like continuing. If not, you've at least fulfilled your commitment to practice at least three exercises every day.

Keeping your word to yourself by practicing every day will strengthen your willpower and protect you from depression. Most of us experience periods of nonclinical depression from time to time, and we are often unaware of what causes these feelings. It is very easy to become irregular in Yoga practice during these times because you may not feel like doing much of anything. Unfortunately, inactivity often just intensifies the depression. Keeping your word to yourself to practice at least three exercises every day will help you avoid this problem.

If on some days you are unable to practice even three exercises, you can still benefit from doing them mentally. Rama told me that just imagining yourself going through the asans with the correct body positions and breath patterns will bring about a beneficial result.

Don't be fooled by the relative simplicity of these warm-up movements. Every exercise in Yoga is a concentrated distillation of effects on the body, breath, and mind. Pay attention to detail: every position of your fingers and toes matters. If the instructions for the exercise do not include any particular focus point for your gaze, look at one spot on the wall or floor to avoid becoming distracted. You can also focus your gaze on the dot in the center of any of the diagrams that are located at the beginning of each chapter.

Watch your breath: in some exercises, you simply let your breath relax into a normal pattern; in others, you coordinate the breath with the movement. Sometimes the breath is held either in or out for a moment. Always breathe through your nose (unless specifically directed to breathe differently), and listen for the steamlike sound that will help you concentrate (see "Five Points for Effective Breathing" in this chapter for more about the sound of the breath).

As with all the exercises in this book, read the instructions thoroughly first so you can do the exercise without having to read the book as you are moving. After you have learned them, the warm-ups will take you two to three minutes.

The Asan Point, included in some of these warm-ups, is the culminating point of the exercise where your body is in position, eyes focused, breath held in or out (depending on the asan), and mind quiet. For more about the Asan Point, see "The Asan Point" in Chapter 1.

1. **Shoulder Roll.** Stand with feet parallel and arms hanging loose at your sides. Lift both shoulders up toward your ears (without bending your elbows) (2.1) and rotate your shoulders in circles, first forward, then backward, at least five times each direction. Keep your arms and hands hanging loosely. Breathe normally.

2. **Neck Stretch.** Be careful with this exercise if you have disk problems in your neck. Gently bend your neck to the right and slightly forward, so your chin reaches down toward your collarbone. Place your left palm on your neck to monitor the stretch. Hold for several seconds, breathing normally (2.2). Repeat on the opposite side.

If you have no neck problems, you may add a Head Rotation: place your hands on your hips or let them hang straight down, and keep your shoulders relaxed. Gently bend your head to the left, bending so your ear is over your shoulder and being careful not to lift your shoulder up. Roll your head forward, chin toward your

chest, and continue rolling your head over toward the right shoulder, then back, then over to the left to complete the circle. Repeat slowly twice more to the left and then three times to the right. Keep shoulders relaxed at all times; the only parts of your body that should move are your head and neck.

3. **Arm Roll.** Stand with feet parallel. Lift your arms straight out to the sides, fingers flexed and palms facing outward (2.3). Maintaining this position, rotate your arms first in large, slow circles and then in small, faster circles. Do each rotation five to eight times in both forward and reverse directions.

2.3

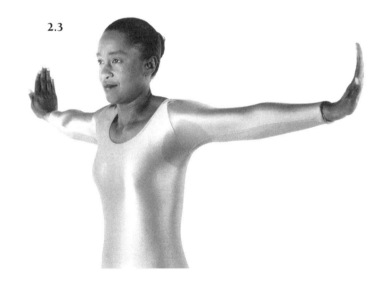

4. **Full Bend.** Stand with feet parallel and arms at your sides. Breathe out completely, then breathe in as you bring your arms up and out to the sides and slightly back, to fully expand your chest (2.4). Now

breathe out as you slowly bend forward, tucking your chin to your chest and reaching down toward the floor (2.5). Keep your knees straight but not locked. If you can reach the floor easily, place your palms flat. If not, just let your arms and hands hang loosely. Let your body relax, holding your breath out. *Asan Point.* Then breathe in as you slowly straighten, bringing your arms up and out to the sides again to repeat the exercise. Repeat three to five times.

5. Full Bend Variation. Stand with feet parallel. Clasp your hands behind you. If you can, press your palms together. For an even greater stretch, lock your elbows so your shoulder blades are squeezed together (2.6). Breathe in and lift your arms in back as far as you can without straining. Breathe out and bend forward, tucking your chin and keeping your arms in position (2.7). Hold your breath out. *Asan Point.* Breathe in and straighten, and repeat the exercise twice more.

2.6

2.4

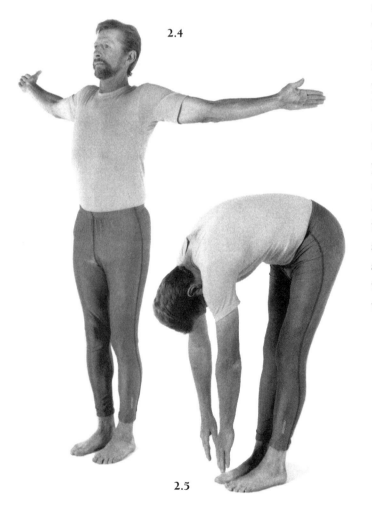

2.5

2.7

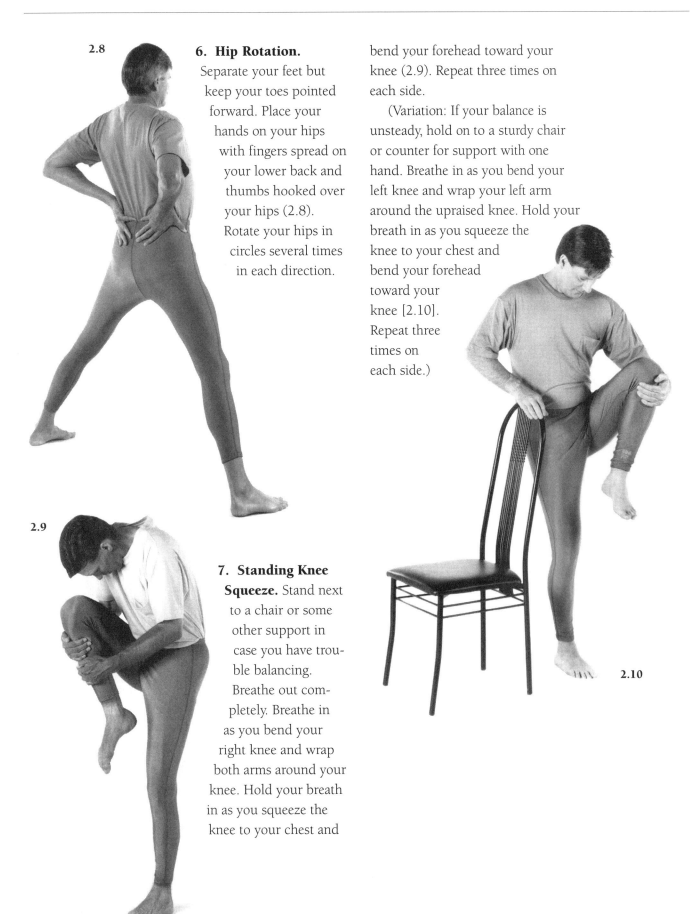

2.8

6. Hip Rotation. Separate your feet but keep your toes pointed forward. Place your hands on your hips with fingers spread on your lower back and thumbs hooked over your hips (2.8). Rotate your hips in circles several times in each direction.

bend your forehead toward your knee (2.9). Repeat three times on each side.

(Variation: If your balance is unsteady, hold on to a sturdy chair or counter for support with one hand. Breathe in as you bend your left knee and wrap your left arm around the upraised knee. Hold your breath in as you squeeze the knee to your chest and bend your forehead toward your knee [2.10]. Repeat three times on each side.)

2.9

7. Standing Knee Squeeze. Stand next to a chair or some other support in case you have trouble balancing. Breathe out completely. Breathe in as you bend your right knee and wrap both arms around your knee. Hold your breath in as you squeeze the knee to your chest and

2.10

Rest Poses

Because the routines in this book are quite vigorous, you will be directed to rest from time to time in one of three positions. Never skip over this step; a rest provides not only physical recovery but also a chance to deepen your experience of the Asan Point. During your rest period, which should last a minimum of thirty seconds, relax your body completely, let your breath return to normal, and try not to think about anything.

2.11

1. **Standing Rest.** Stand with your feet a few inches apart. Keep your legs straight, but do not lock your knees. Close your eyes and try to balance equally on both feet. Let your arms relax at your sides (2.11). Imagine a string at the top of your head keeping your head and body straight but relaxed. Let your breath relax and hold the position for several seconds.

2. **Baby Pose.** Kneel and sit on your feet. Bend forward, keeping your hips on your feet, so your forehead or the top of your head rests on the floor. Bring your arms to your sides and let your elbows fall outward slightly so that your shoulders relax completely (2.12). Breathe naturally and relax your entire body.

Hold for as long as you can comfortably. If you cannot bend completely forward while keeping your hips on your feet due to a large midsection or stiff knees or hips, just bend as far forward as you can. It's more important to try to keep your hips on your heels than to rest your head on the floor. If you have high blood pressure, or if placing your head lower than your heart is uncomfortable, rest your head on folded arms on a pillow in front of you (2.13), but try to keep your hips on your feet. If your knees or hips are too stiff for this position, place a pillow under your hips as well (2.14).

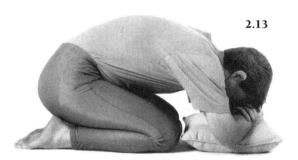

2.12

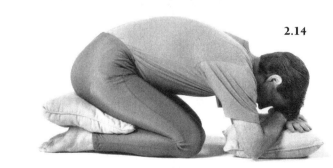

2.13

2.14

3. Corpse Pose. Lie on your back on your mat with legs together and arms at your sides (2.15). Do not place a pillow under your head

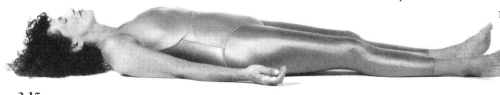

2.15

(unless necessary for medical reasons), because you want to avoid pressure on the veins and nerves at the back of the neck. If your lower back feels tense, place a pillow under your thighs just above your knees. Close your eyes and let all parts of your body sink into the floor and relax. Especially check your eyes, jaw, shoulders, and stomach. Let your breath relax. Hold this rest position for at least one minute, or until your breath returns to normal and your body feels completely relaxed. Try to relax so much that you no longer even feel the floor.

quieting and concentrating effects of breathing techniques done just prior to meditation. In this chapter you will learn several breathing techniques that will strengthen your respiratory system, improve concentration and willpower, stabilize your metabolism, and energize the subtle pathways of the body.

My teacher Lakshmanjoo talked a lot about the importance of breathing. He said that the most important point is awareness: to continually watch the breath when breathing in, when breathing out, and at the turning point of the breath. He said that watching your breath in this manner is most effective if you can do it not just during your regular daily period of Yoga practice, but in every action of your life, such as while walking, talking, and so on.

The body of the person practicing the regulation of breath becomes harmoniously developed, emits sweet scent, and looks beautiful and lovely.

(Siva Samhita)

Breathing Techniques

In Yoga, the breath, body, and mind are like a three-legged stool. Without all three legs, you will fall over. Many people who practice Yoga skip over breathing techniques, thinking that they are less important than the exercises or meditation. In fact, correct breathing is what makes the Yoga exercises complete and effective, and meditation is greatly assisted by the

POSITIONS FOR BREATHING

Before you start learning the breathing techniques, you must find a seated position that you can hold comfortably for five to ten minutes. If you prefer to sit cross-legged on the floor, sit on one or two cushions to raise your hips and take the strain off your lower back (2.16). This position, with one heel in front of the other, is called the Perfect Pose. You can test your limberness by noting whether your hips are higher than your knees

2.16

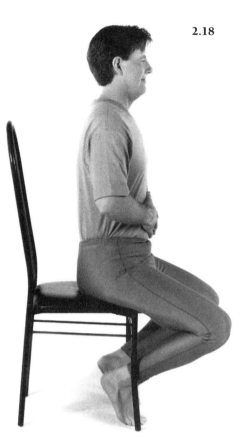

2.18

2.17

when you sit cross-legged; if your knees are higher, you will not be able to hold the position very long without experiencing back strain.

If you can't find a comfortable cross-legged position, try sitting in a kneeling position with a small cushion under your ankles or between your ankles and hips. You can also straddle a pile of cushions (2.17), or even sit on the edge of a chair (2.18). In a chair, tuck your toes under to get that same slant from hips to knees, and don't lean against the back of the chair. You can also practice many breathing techniques leaning against a wall with a pillow behind your lower back to keep your back straight, or lying on your back on the floor or on a firm bed. Do not use a pillow under your head.

FIVE POINTS FOR EFFECTIVE BREATHING

1. Always breathe through your nose.
2. Maintain an erect posture with your head balanced straight on your neck; do not tilt your head forward or back.
3. Make a steamlike sound with your breath—the sound of air hitting the back of your throat first instead of the inside of your nos-

trils. This will give you greater control over the length of the breath, and will also serve as an aid to focusing. To make this sound, think about relaxing the muscles around your nose and drawing the air in from the back of your throat instead. If the sound still eludes you, whisper *Ha*, then close your mouth and make the same sound.

4. If you notice yourself feeling dizzy, stop the breathing exercise for a few minutes until the dizziness goes away, then begin again. Usually this happens when you are first beginning to learn to breathe and goes away after a week or two.

5. A set of wax earplugs (such as swimmers use) can help you concentrate and also help dampen outside noises that might distract you.

COMPLETE BREATH

The *Complete Breath* is a diaphragmatic breath pattern. Start by placing your hands on your belly just below your navel. Breathe out completely; you should feel your hands move inward as your belly contracts. Push in with your hands and tighten your belly muscles to accentuate the contraction (2.19). Now breathe in, release your belly muscles, and feel your hands move outward as the breath fills the bottom part of your lungs and expands the diaphragm (2.20). Pretend that the air is filling your entire belly. Always breathe through your nose and concentrate on the steamlike sound of your breath.

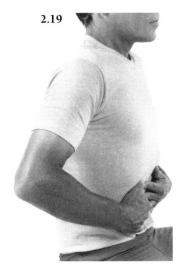

2.19

2.20

The Complete Breath starts with this movement and then extends the air into the top portions of the lungs. When you breathe in, you expand first the belly, then your ribs, then your chest. When you breathe out, you let the chest relax first, then the ribs, and finally contract the belly to expel the last of the air. Breathe in from the bottom up; breathe out from the top down.

When you are comfortable with the movements of the Complete Breath, turn your attention toward the length of the breath. In the Complete Breath, the inhalation and exhalation should be equal. Most people can naturally breathe out longer than they breathe in; in this case, you may need to temporarily shorten your exhalation to match your inhalation. You can measure your breath by counting or by watching the second hand of a clock, but try not to count the entire time. After you've established a comfortable pattern, close your eyes and try to empty your mind of everything except the sound of the breath.

Start with five to ten repetitions of the Complete Breath at least once a day.

ALTERNATE NOSTRIL BREATH

The main purpose of this breathing technique is to balance the two halves of the body and the two aspects of the personality (see "Balancing Both Halves of the Personality" in Chapter 8).

In a comfortable seated position or in a chair, curl the first and second fingers of your right hand inward, holding them down with the fleshy part of your thumb. The third and fourth fingers should remain extended. Close your right nostril with your thumb (2.21), and breathe in through the left nostril only. Close the left nostril with your third and fourth fingers (2.22), open the right, and breathe out, then in again, through the right nostril. Continue alternating by breathing out, then in, through one side at a time. Repeat five to ten times.

If one side of your nose is blocked, try this technique for opening it: If the right side is blocked, place your right fist in your left armpit and hold for a few minutes until the right side opens. Reverse the procedure to open the opposite side.

Another method is to simply lie on your side for a few minutes: if the right nostril is blocked, lie on your *left* side.

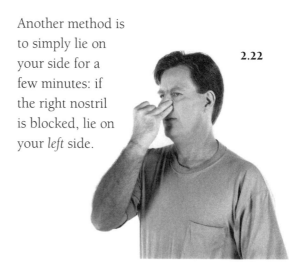

2.22

THE COOLING BREATH

This technique has a cooling effect on the body; it also improves resistance to disease and enhances physical beauty.

In a comfortable seated position or in a chair, breathe out completely. Extend your tongue and curl the sides in (2.23) and breathe in slowly. Exhale with mouth closed. Make the inhalation and exhalation equal in length. Repeat five to ten times.

2.21

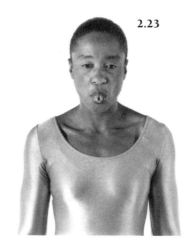

2.23

SOFT BELLOWS BREATH

This exercise tones and relaxes the muscles and nerves involved in respiration. It is an excellent preparatory technique for meditation because it focuses the mind very quickly. Its Sanskrit name, *Kapalabhati*, literally means *shining skull*, which refers to the power of this technique to stimulate the movement of energy of kundalini to the top of the head. In mythical language this implies that a lotus is opening at the top of the head.

Sit comfortably in a cross-legged position with your hips raised on cushions, or sit on the edge of a chair with feet tucked under slightly. Place one hand on your diaphragm (the soft triangular area just below your ribs) to monitor the movement (2.24). This breathing technique has two parts. The first is a gentle bellows-like movement of the diaphragm—*not* the belly. Start breathing in and out fairly quickly—about one cycle of inhalation/exhalation per second—but evenly. In other words, don't emphasize either inhalation or exhalation. In order to allow this short, fast breath to move smoothly, you will need to *reverse* the instructions given for all other breathing and exercise techniques about making the steamlike sound that originates at the back of the throat. For the bellows technique, relax your throat so you feel the breath mostly at the tips of your nostrils instead of the back of your throat.

Start with only ten repetitions of the bellows, then for the second part of this exercise, breathe out completely (revert to the back-of-the-throat sound now). Breathe in completely, hold your breath in for about three seconds, then breathe out very slowly until all your breath is out. Then relax and breathe normally for several seconds.

Repeat the entire sequence—ten bellows, full short exhalation, full short inhalation, very long exhalation, relaxed breath—three to five times.

When the breath is suspended then the thinking mind also is suspended. . . . When the mind is absorbed, breathing subsides; when the power of breath subsides, the mind is also absorbed in stillness. . . . When mind and breath are absorbed in each other, the immeasurable joy of samadhi *(absorption) ensues.*
(Hatha Yoga Pradipika)

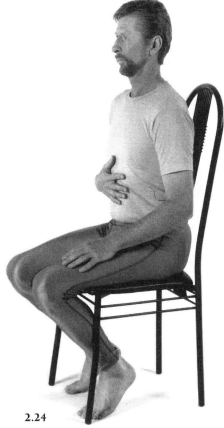

2.24

THE RISING BREATH

This exercise creates a wonderful brightness of mind. It increases the heat of the body and contributes to better health and greater strength.

In a seated position on the floor or in a chair, grasp your knees firmly with both hands. Breathe in completely, then breathe out completely. Hold your breath out, tuck your chin into the hollow of your collarbone, and pull your stomach muscles in and up (2.25). Relax your stomach, then continue holding your breath as you pull in your stomach, relax, pull in, and relax a third time. Now relax your stomach and slowly breathe in. Continue breathing in and out a few times to rest. Each repetition includes three contractions with the breath held out. Start with three repetitions.

2.25

Relaxation and Meditation

Many years ago, I was hired to teach a Yoga class in a city on the East Coast. When I arrived at the site, I was hospitably ushered into a room exotically draped in silk cloths, with fans to move the drapes, a music system, and strobe lights thoughtfully placed near the place where I would sit. My hosts asked me to sit so I could see the effects of the lights and music as background for the meditation class. I sat. The effects were turned on, and I must admit it was lovely. The undulating drapes and the lights and mood music created quite a dreamy atmosphere. However, I had to explain to my hosts as diplomatically as I could that this was not a suitable background for meditative practice.

When you practice meditation, give yourself as much environmental silence and solitude as possible. Go into a room where you can be completely alone, close the door, turn off the telephone, and keep out the pets. Ask others in the household to leave you undisturbed for fifteen to thirty minutes. This may be difficult at first if you believe that you must always be available for others. Try to approach this meditation period thinking, "This is time only for myself—nothing else. It is a time to repair and refill the resources of my inner self. It's time to put water back into my own well."

When you are really relaxed and trying to withdraw from thought, you need a protected area where nothing can startle you. Loud noises such as bells ringing or doors slamming can be extremely upsetting. If you live on a busy street or in a noisy household, the wax earplugs mentioned earlier in this chapter can be very useful. If you are lucky enough to reach some depth of silence, an abrupt change of consciousness can be harmful. It could make you jittery and cross all day, and even bring on a headache or unwell feelings. You must be careful to emerge from the silence of your meditation slowly and carefully, bringing your mind and body back into normal consciousness in a protected way. When you have given yourself three to five minutes to resume your natural activities, you will feel much better, steady and rested.

Ideally, your meditation period should follow your exercise and breathing routine. If you don't have time to practice all three parts at one time, try at least to end your exercise segment with a few minutes of complete relaxation. Use the "Quick Relaxation," lying on your mat, and rest for a few minutes. Then practice your breathing techniques and a longer meditation at another time of day.

MEDITATION POSITIONS

If you are a beginner, or if you have very stiff hips or knees, meditate lying on your back on your mat in the Corpse Pose. If you are comfortable in a cross-legged or kneeling position and are able to sit with your back straight, you may meditate that way. Never force yourself to sit upright if your knees, hips, or back are feeling any discomfort; the point in meditation is to *not* think about your body for a few minutes, and an uncomfortable position can be overwhelmingly distracting.

In a seated position, your back will be most comfortable if you lift your hips a few inches with cushions. Place your feet so that the heels line up together: this is called the Perfect Pose (2.16). If you can sit in a Lotus Pose (see Chapter 6) or a Half Lotus (one foot on top of the opposite thigh and the other foot tucked underneath the thigh), you can meditate that way, but be sure you can sit for twenty to thirty minutes without strain.

If your knees and hips are too stiff for a cross-legged position, you can sit against a wall with legs outstretched or in a straight chair, with a pillow behind your lower back for support (2.26). The most important point is to be comfortable. To limber your hips and knees faster, practice the Fatigue Routine (see Chapter 4) at least four times a week, and sit cross-legged at home whenever you think of it; for instance, while reading or watching television.

Wear socks for meditation, and wrap yourself in a blanket or shawl. When you slip into meditation, your body temperature will drop, and the uncomfortable feeling will intrude into your thoughts, keeping you from real silence. Meditation is a very

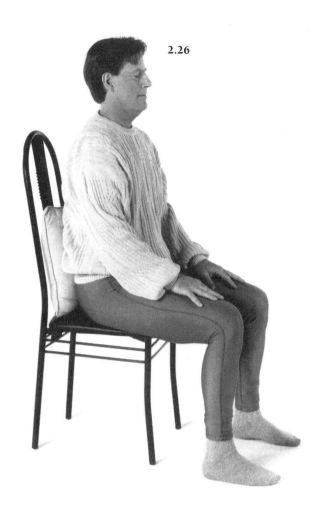

2.26

vulnerable time, because you are so quiet. An extra wrap adds a sort of psychic feeling of protection during this inner-directed period.

QUICK RELAXATION

Use this technique when you have only a few minutes in which to relax.

Start by lying on your back on your mat, with legs a few inches apart and arms at your sides, palms facing up. All at once, tighten all the muscles of your body and lift up so you are balancing on your buttocks. Then release and let your body fall

back to the floor. Shake each limb in turn: left arm, right arm, left leg, right leg. Roll your head gently from side to side. Shake your entire body gently and feel the sensation of melting into the floor. Take a deep, slow breath in, then release it all at once and relax your breath. With your eyes closed, rest for a few minutes, or go on to the meditation instructions.

This technique can be done at any other time of day as well—even while sitting at your desk or in your car.

COMPLETE RELAXATION

In this relaxation procedure, you will take five to ten minutes relaxing each part of your body individually. The purpose of this exercise is not only to relax your body completely but also to begin focusing your mind. As you move your attention from one part to the other, your mind will slow down and rest, so that by the time you are ready to go into meditation, your inner conversation will have lessened.

Take the position you have chosen for meditation. It's better not to move after the relaxation process, so you can slip right into meditation afterward. If you begin in a seated position, however, lie down at any time if you become uncomfortable.

Lying Down Position. Lie on your back on your mat, wearing socks and with a shawl or sweater over you. If your mat is not large enough for your entire body to fit, be sure your head is resting on it. Your back should be straight but not tense. If your lower back feels tense, place a cushion under your knees. Do not use a pillow under your head; this might cause pressure on the veins and nerves in the back of the neck, which would affect your meditation. Keep your legs together, and place your arms at your sides close in to your body, with the palms of your hands facing up. Your fingers will be slightly curled.

Seated Position. Find a comfortable seated position, whether cross-legged on the floor or with your back leaning against the wall, or seated in a chair. There is a natural small curve at the small of the back. If you feel tension anywhere in your back, add a pillow under your hips and, if you are leaning against a sturdy surface, place a pillow at your lower back. Let your hands rest comfortably on your knees or in your lap. There is no need to hold your hands in any special position. Wear socks and wrap a sweater or shawl around you (2.27).

Begin by closing your eyes and picturing your body. Imagine it surrounded by a transparent shell of very still air that moves only slightly with your breath. As you go through the relaxation sequence, try to relax each part of your body *without moving it.*

Bring your attention to your forehead and relax it. Imagine soft fingers smoothing out any lines in your forehead from the inside. Relax your eyes. Think about how they look, as if you were looking into a mirror. Let the lids become heavy, and relax even your eyelashes. Relax all the many

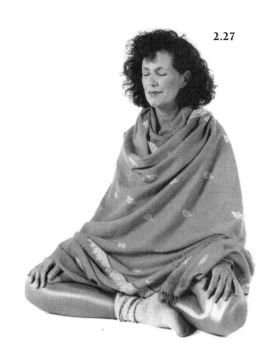

2.27

muscles around your eyes, so it feels as if your eyes are sinking into your face. Then imagine soft fingers inside your face smoothing your cheeks. Relax the corners of your mouth, and let your jaw relax. Feel your teeth become so relaxed that they feel loose. Let your ears relax back.

Bring your attention slowly down to your neck. Feel the muscles in your neck *from the inside,* and relax them. Let your voice box slacken. Smooth your collarbones, and gently let your shoulders sink into the floor and rest. Think about the structure of your shoulder joint, and loosen it in your mind. You don't have to move your arms for a few minutes. Relax your arms, starting with the upper arm, then the elbow, then the forearm, and finally your wrists and hands. Imagine yourself sitting next to a small stream of clear, cool water in the mountains. Listen to the water gently flowing by, then dip your hands into the water and just let them float, fingers curled just like a baby's hands when it sleeps.

Now slowly bring your attention back up your arms into your chest. Imagine your heart. Picture it strong, healthy, and relaxed. While you are picturing your heart, take a deep, slow breath in, and relax your heart as you let the air out all at once in a deep sigh. Feel your ribs relaxing, and all the muscles in between the ribs. Picture your lungs, take another deep, slow breath in, filling your lungs, then release it, sigh the breath out, and then let your breath go back to normal.

Imagine your stomach and all your internal organs. Picture everything working perfectly and resting. Relax your hipbones and the joint between your hips and thighs. Let your thighs fall toward the floor and relax. Now imagine your knees. Try to picture the complex structure of your knees, and then relax them.

Relax your calves and ankles, and then picture your feet. Imagine your toes, and the soles of your feet. Let your feet fall outward and relax them. Imagine standing in that cool stream of clear water. Look at your toes under the water and feel the current flowing over your feet.

Now move your attention to your heels and ankles. Relax the tendon behind your heels and move up the back of your legs, relaxing them again. Relax the base of your spine. Visualize your spine in a gentle curve, the vertebrae strong, healthy, and straight, and the spinal cord like a shining conduit of electricity running up inside. Starting at the base of your spine, relax each vertebra and the muscles and nerves that surround it. Relax your shoulder blades, then the back of your neck. Feel the spot where your spine joins into your skull, and relax it. Let the bones of your skull separate slightly in your mind, and picture your brain resting inside, gently floating.

Now bring your attention back to your forehead and check to make sure that your face and body are completely relaxed. Visualize liquid gold flowing throughout your body as you begin to meditate.

A MASTER'S OUTLOOK ON MEDITATION

Lakshmanjoo once wrote that the state of concentration required for meditation can be achieved if the student's mind is free from all "domestic worries," all daily routine activities are completed, and after a full amount of sleep. He said the mind must be absolutely free from all preoccupations in order to meditate "without deviation and see inside yourself." As you can see, this is an impossible condition of most people's minds. I have found great success in suggesting that you simply stop all thought for as long as you can. If thought patterns continue to disturb you, simply repeat the process of stopping thought. Discontinue talking to yourself in your mind.

The following is an excerpt from a conversation I had with Lakshmanjoo several years ago on the subject of meditation. I include it here to give you a master's outlook on meditation:

Alice: Swamiji, what is the result of that steady directing of your thoughts—what is the pinnacle?

Lakshmanjoo: The ultimate point is thoughtless point. You have to tread on the path of thought towards thoughtless point. Thoughtless point is the aim that we are to achieve.

Alice: Could you say that that would be silence?

Lakshmanjoo: Yes, but this is not absolute silence. This is silence in movement. Steadiness in movement. Thought in thoughtless state.

Alice: That would be an awareness of a thoughtless state, wouldn't it, Swamiji?

Lakshmanjoo: So, it means that this whole universe is without thought. If we try to realize it, this will be thoughtless—nothing is in movement. Although everything seems to be in movement, it is not moving.

Alice: What makes it move then?

Lakshmanjoo: It is one-pointed, it *seems* only.

Alice: It *seems* to move—

Lakshmanjoo: Through ignorance. If you come to realize it properly, this movement will end in stability. There will be no movement. So this is unmoving movement, this whole universe, and that is God, that is God.

Alice: Time changes, then, doesn't it, Swamiji?

Lakshmanjoo: Time is only a collection of works. If there is no work to do, there is no time. If there is nowhere to go, there is no space. And space and time only exist when there are things to be done.

Alice: So, it could be an invention of the mind?

Lakshmanjoo: Yes.

Alice: Swamiji, does this mean you are centering yourself?

Lakshmanjoo: Yes, this is centering. This is real centering. (from *Conversations with Swami Lakshmanjoo, Volume I: Aspects of Kashmir Shaivism* [see Appendix C])

You can see how difficult the process is in reality! Meditation is not something that you master instantly; it is a process that takes quite a period of time.

YOUR MEDITATION SESSION

Start your meditation period by thinking of the sound *Om*. This word is a mantram—a sound formula that has a specific effect on the mind when it is repeated or listened to. The diagram at the beginning of this chapter is a representation of the sound *Om*, which is said to reside in the forehead. *Om* is actually composed of three sounds: *A*, *U*, and *M*, which can be thought of as three states of consciousness. The sound *A*, which is pronounced with the mouth open, is said to represent the waking state, when we are most open to the external world. The sound *U*, pronounced with a partially closed mouth, is said to represent the dreaming state, when we are asleep but our mind is still active. The sound *M* is pronounced with closed mouth and is said to represent the state of deep sleep, when we are not conscious of the external world. The silence before and after the word may be viewed as the silence of meditation, also called *turiya*, or the fourth state.

The mantram *Om* is repeated before meditation because it helps you to focus on stillness. If you use my meditation cassette (see Appendix C) I sing the mantram to you before and after the meditation session. You do not need to sing *Om* out loud; just repeat it several times silently to yourself, and then let the sound fade away into silence. Gently try to maintain that silence for as long as you can. When you notice your mind leaping after a thought, finish the thought and then let it go away. Notice the feeling of silence after the thought leaves your mind, and see how long you can observe that silence before another thought comes by to attract your attention.

Meditate for at least fifteen minutes; thirty is ideal. Instead of setting an alarm, which would startle you out of your stillness, tell yourself before you start how long you want to stay in meditation, and your mind will automatically start to come back to normal consciousness after that time. Always give yourself three to five minutes to fully return to your normal activity levels after meditation. Leaping out of meditation can cause extreme nervousness and sensitivity; the transition should be very slow. After your meditation session, continue sitting or lying in your meditation position for five minutes if you can, remembering what happened during your meditation session and trying not to judge it as "good" or "bad." Then, when you feel like moving, slowly stretch your arms and legs and take a deep breath, then let it out. Enjoy the relaxed feeling of body and mind.

Think of your meditation period as a time to heal stress. In Yoga philosophy, stress is defined as two things attracting each other; in meditation, the two things that attract each other are a thought and your attention. Every time a thought appears to you, your mind is attracted to it. When that thought leaves, there may be a moment or two of silence—but soon another thought appears, and your mind turns toward the new thought. This is a picture of inner stress operating. Usually we think of the word *stress* as having a negative connotation. From this explanation, you can see that in Yoga meditation the term *stress* merely refers to this movement of attraction in the mind; it is neither negative nor positive. The more the mind leaps to thought, the more stress you are experiencing. The purpose of meditation is to reduce that constant movement so you can experience silence.

Usually, this constant stress of mental engagement with thoughts goes unnoticed; all day long our minds are in continual conversation. With regular practice of meditation, you will begin to notice the activity that goes on in your mind and, as your practices become steadier, you will experience small periods of complete silence in your meditation. Although these moments are small and fleeting at first, you will feel a definite relief from stress. When you finish your meditation practice for the day, you will feel rested and refreshed.

This is a far different experience from simply replacing the sounds and patterns in the mind with other sounds and patterns reproduced by music, lights, or in some cases, alcohol or drugs. The actual product of silence in the mind gives a complete rest to both your mental and physical systems.

The biggest obstacle for most students is their continual internal conversation. In order to experience meditation, all inner talk must stop. Try to think nothing. Your mind will jump to its attraction; when you notice this, gently go back to thinking nothing. Beware of judging yourself, saying, "Oh, I had a good meditation" or "I had a bad meditation." Meditation is simply a matter of slow, steady withdrawal from a constant pattern of attraction of thought. This takes practice. There is no "good" or "bad" in meditation; the important thing is that you put in your time every day.

Meditation is a feeling of watching inside your head; there is no conversation and nothing to see, yet you continue to watch. In the terms of the philosophy of Kashmir Shaivism, this type of meditation practice leads to the experience of "delight, wonder, and astonishment" as you begin to realize that there is something else, beyond your normal perception, lying in that silence, which you can begin to observe. Usually, it happens with shocking clarity when you are off guard, not looking for or demanding any response. Suddenly a brilliant response of silence will be experienced, as if meditation is reaching toward you, instead of you exerting the effort. When this happens, you know you have begun to experience meditative practice. You will have felt the silence.

3
Fantasy

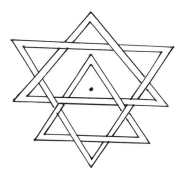

Source of creation floating in the cosmic waters; the
union of the male and female principles of personality

Fantasy is viewed by many people as a pleasant—but useless—pastime in which we all occasionally indulge. Children especially slip happily into fantasy as they grow and play. In childhood many hopes and problems are worked out in fantasy before they are lived; the common phenomenon of giving a doll a personality is a way of practicing interactions and working out anxieties. Many children have imaginary friends who are quite real to them and who help them negotiate the fearful process of growing up. If you spend much time with children, you will notice that when free indulgence in fantasy is allowed, boredom, depression, and poor self-image are much less apparent.

Unfortunately, the retreat to fantasy is often discouraged as we get older. This simple, useful tool is viewed as impractical, and is usually trained out of us at an early age. Unless you have studied acting or other arts, your exposure to the use of fantasy has probably been limited to getting "lost" in a movie or book, or the idle daydreams that we all indulge in when our minds are not busy. Throughout the ages, however, Yoga has celebrated the use of fantasy as a basic force of change; Yoga teaches and uses fantasy in all forms of practice. Yoga philosophy states that fantasy is the bridge to the unconscious; when we strengthen and support that bridge, we are no longer separate from the hidden side of our nature.

Fantasy brings relief from the ordinary, everyday thought that is often so stressful. Most of us are always thinking about something, and usually there are strong feelings associated with every thought. Our minds experience a constant barrage of reaction and anxiety that is very stressful because it seems to perpetuate a separation between the self (subject) and what the self is considering (object). This instability of separation is what causes stressful feelings. Fantasy corrects this problem by allowing you to enjoy several states of consciousness at one time. When the stress of separateness is reduced, you are able to experience what is called in Kashmir Shaivism "delight, wonder, and astonishment." In other words, fantasy opens up the immense possibilities of a complete consciousness that gives you constant support, because you realize that you are resting on something that doesn't move. Fantasy has been called the "perfect experience" for this very reason.

According to Yogic thought, you always have the ability to experience many possible states of consciousness. Fantasy teaches you how to observe them. You never again need be a prisoner of unwanted thought, which often leads to depression, boredom, or upset. This state of limitless choice is described in the *Isa Upanishad* as "the all which wants nothing; for there is nothing to the all which it can want." You experience a state of fullness, where feelings of separateness evaporate.

DESPAIR, DEPRESSION, AND BOREDOM

Fantasy techniques are quite helpful in dealing with the pervasive problems of despair, depression, and boredom—feelings that hang like a dark cloud around individuals who think they are trapped and have no choice. These individuals become slaves in a type of consciousness that seems to be a long, narrow road of doing things they do not want to do, with no end in sight.

These modes of suffering have one important thing in common: the sufferer truly believes that relief can come only through the auspices of someone or something outside the self. In other words, if you suffer from any of these problems, you have to go somewhere, or have the money to buy something, or depend on someone other than yourself to open the door of the prison in which you are trapped. In most cases, these three bears of existence—despair, depression, and boredom—can follow you no matter how far you go or how much you are willing to spend, and sometimes they even place themselves between you and any other person who might try to help you be free of them. They are indeed the true qualities of separateness.

People who practice Yoga seriously eventually come to realize that the power to be comfortable with these seemingly ever-present qualities lies within themselves. Yoga asans, breathing, meditation, and fantasy techniques done regularly, even in very small time periods of fifteen to twenty minutes a day, accompanied by attention to the ethical guidelines discussed elsewhere in this book (see Chapter 6), can easily help you choose a fresh, free existence. You will realize that there is no need to use destructive behavior to escape, nor even any need to beg assistance from friends or family. The answer lies in realizing that you have a choice, and this realization comes only from steady practice. It comes from within. New pathways of communication open inside you, allowing a fresh approach to what seemed to be an inflexible position. This does not provide a permanent vacation from these burdensome qualities, but it does offer an ability to remain balanced while they are functioning, bringing a relief from the trapped feeling.

In many cases, even when external help is offered, people trapped in these feelings are unable to accept it because this change would push them beyond the limits of their present fantasy of themselves. Yoga practice can enlarge and enhance your fantasy of yourself so that you have room to expand and move and eventually become able to choose to move toward relief. Fantasy is the key to this necessary type of expansion.

Fantasy is the basic training of Tantric Yoga, a type of Yoga experience that recognizes the value of all the world's manifestations (as opposed to more traditional forms of Yoga such as Vedanta, which are sometimes predicated on the rejection of the body and the everyday world). In Tantric thought, the body is the most perfect and powerful of all *yantras* (diagrams of emotional power); thus the performance of Yoga asans itself becomes an expression of Tantra. You are never urged to a cold asceticism, which would require severing the links to life, but instead you can welcome a gathering up of existence into your own being.

The knowledge and power of our own being is designed and supported first in fantasy—then it takes form in reality. Just as you have to think a word before you speak or write it, the entire world of names and forms, according to Tantra, originates in fantasy. According to this theory, every moment you create yourself anew from your fantasy picture of yourself. In order to grow and change, your fantasy of yourself must also change. Many times I have seen people stuck in an image of themselves at some important time in their lives. Outwardly, it seems as if they have moved on, but internally, they are caught in an earlier image of themselves that they are unable to let go of. For instance, recently a student wrote me that his formerly well-behaved thirteen-year-old son was beginning to exhibit behavior problems. This man couldn't understand what had gone wrong. I immediately saw that this father was unable to let go of his own fantasy of his son's life and consequently was unable to allow the boy to develop his own fantasy. Unconsciously, the boy felt this restriction and was acting against it.

Many years ago, I discovered that students who face and deal with their desires and fears in fantasy, while supporting themselves with daily Yoga exercises, meditation, and a proper diet, become much stronger and are able to allow their lives to change and develop in very satisfying ways. In this chapter I offer two very effective fantasy techniques that will put you in touch with your inner self and allow you to bring the two halves of yourself together.

The "Hall of Space": A Fantasy Technique

This technique is helpful in examining the everyday concerns that remain uppermost in your mind and prevent you from becoming quiet in meditation. Individual desires and fears are so varied that it would be impossible to address each one individually. This fantasy technique allows a great variety of problems and issues to be addressed with a single method.

Lie down on your back on your mat in the Corpse Pose with your arms at your sides, legs together, and eyes closed. Don't use a pillow behind your head. You can also do this exercise sitting in a chair as long as your back is straight. Stay warm. Go through a complete relaxation of your body as described in Chapter 2.

Begin your fantasy exercise by bringing your inner vision of attention to your forehead. Pretend that you are looking down a long hallway. There are several doors leading off this central hallway—some to the left, some to the right. Picture the hallway in every detail: the color of the walls, whether there is carpet or tile or wood on the floor, the color of the doors, the type of hardware on the doors, the lighting in the hallway—all the small details that you can invent in your fantasy. Make it complete in your mind before you enter it.

Now take a most important step: cover your entire body with armor. Imagine the most beautiful, heroic armor you can create. Pay attention to all of the details, such as the color and weight of the armor, the type of helmet and gloves, the boots, and the fasteners. Then, when your body is completely protected with armor, create a beautiful sword of your own design and take it in your hand.

The reason for the protection of this armor and sword is simple: In fantasy you are exploring the unknown world of your unconscious. Although everything you will find there is part of you, much of it will be unfamiliar, and some things might even be frightening at first. The conscious mind often feels anxiety about the unknown; the symbolic protection of the armor and sword that you create in your mind lets you observe your fantasy world without fear.

When your armor and sword are firmly in place, imagine that you are entering the hallway. Choose one of the doors, put your hand on the knob, and open it. Stand protected by all your armor and your sword, and simply observe what is there in that room. Realize that you can step back and shut the door anytime you wish. I suggest that at first you try to observe for about a minute before leaving the room. When you decide to leave, shut the door, walk back to the entrance of the hall, carefully remove your armor, and observe yourself resting in the Corpse Pose. Give yourself plenty of time to change your physical orientation from the fantasy experience back to resting. Then, think about what happened and carefully evaluate what you have discovered.

You can put names on the various doors in your hallway according to what concerns are uppermost in your mind when you try to meditate. Some examples are fear, illness, anxiety about a confrontation, difficulty in a relationship, pressure at work, and so on. If you have a specific problem that continually bothers you in daily thought or in meditation, create a special room in your fantasy exercise for it. Put its name on one of the doors, and after you put on your armor and walk down the hall, simply open the door and look in. You don't have to enter; you only want to observe. When you have had enough, close the door and walk away. Always remember to put on your armor and your sword before entering the hallway.

If you are beginning this technique for the first time, the following questions and topics can provide some structure to get you started. Use these to name the doors in your hallway until you think of other issues you'd like to explore. Do not try to do all the doorways in one session; one at a time is enough! Try a new one each week. You will notice that most of the suggestions for door names seem to be about fears or other thoughts that might most disturb your meditation. You can add any subject or feeling that you like and put that name on a door in your hallway. Many of my students have especially enjoyed putting the name "love" on one of the doors; the results are usually very interesting.

1. What is your biggest physical fear?
2. What object are you most afraid of losing?
3. What makes you happiest?
4. What person are you most afraid of losing?
5. What person do you dislike or fear the most?
6. In the next week, what event do you dread the most?
7. Do you feel unnamed or non-specific fear? (Use "unknown" on the door.)

After you have put names on the doors of your hallway, notice whether the doors of greatest importance to you are on the right or the left side of the hall. The right and left doors signify the Apollonian and Dionysian personalities, respectively (see "Balancing Both Halves of the Personality" in Chapter 8). It will be interesting for you to see how many doors of each personality you are able to use.

In the beginning, try to practice this technique just before meditation. After you have done it a few times, you will be able to go through the whole routine in five minutes or less. You will notice that quieting your mind in meditation will be much easier after this practice.

Sometimes students quit in frustration, saying that they never see anything when they open the doors in their mind. Usually I find that these people are afraid to try, indicating that the obstacle confronting them in meditation is very difficult. If you find yourself in this position, simply continue with the fantasy exercise until you begin to enjoy some success. If there is something

in your mind, eventually you will be able to see it. Probably you have never attempted to see it or communicate with it before. Even if you open the door and nothing is there at first, if you continue to do the technique, something will appear. I have never known a student who didn't eventually find something behind the door.

If you practice this technique daily, you will experience great improvement in your concentration and your ability to deal with daily problems. Most of all, however, regular practice of this exercise allows the hidden, unseen experience that lies within you to emerge. It is no longer something that is just felt; it takes shape, and you are fully protected to deal with it as you wish. When you have mastered the technique, you will find that you can use it as an immediate solution to whatever draws your mind away from the silence of meditation. It has a great clarifying effect. You will no longer wander around saying "Something is bothering me but I don't know what it is." You can discover what it is and start to deal with it safely.

THE VALUE OF STUDY: AN EXPERIENCE OF EXPANSION

He who contemplates on sunya *(void or vacuum or space) while walking or standing or dreaming or waking becomes altogether ethereal, and is absorbed in the* chid akasha *(the ether of pure consciousness).*

(Siva Samhita)

If you are serious about progressing in Yoga, it is a good idea to spend some time each day—in addition to your practice of asans, breathing, and meditation—reading and studying books that are related to your interest in Yoga. Ancient and modern texts on Yoga, philosophy, world religions, mythology—choose whatever subject interests you. Study should be a happy pastime, and it will allow for expansion in fantasy and thought. The problem of finding oneself is addressed in all literature, and you can vicariously enjoy seeing yourself as the main character trying to find himself or herself. Many times, the images that will illuminate your fantasy techniques will be archetypal images, and your study will allow you to refer to these images historically and poetically.

Even though you may not immediately understand what you are reading, you will often experience a new and intense feeling when you read. It is like the feeling you have when, for instance, you are walking on a beach, looking at the constantly changing waves, or gazing at the sky at night, when it is filled with endless diagrams of stars. For a moment at these times, your normal daily thought stops, and your mind expands into the vast unknown regions. You can actually feel yourself expand as you escape from the norm and are drawn into the void of space or light. Such feelings often become quite sweet and precious to us. This expansive feeling in daily practice is needed for the practice of Yoga. It allows room for concepts and ideas that you do not normally use.

Most people believe that these types of experiences happen only in such quiet, solitary interludes, but the Yoga student learns that these feelings of expansion and unity are always there, whether you are walking in the woods or working at your desk. This type of experience allows you to work without stress because your creativity can flow with expansion, unblocked. Blocked creativity creates stress.

Training the body to become strong and fit then becomes a stepping-stone, a strong support for this expansion. Your practice goes far beyond "bending and breathing"; in fact, the strength of your body becomes the support vehicle for this new experience. The relationship between corporeal and spiritual becomes solidified as you become more comfortable with the unknown, creative parts of yourself.

When you were a child, you probably sat on the lap of your parent or grandparent while he or she told you stories. You felt protected and supported while you explored the world in fantasy through their stories. This is a valuable experience, because it teaches you to move comfortably into fantasy without self-destruction or fear. Supported fantasy leads to happy, fearless expansion of the mind and spirit.

When we have a transcendent experience, our first impulse is to try to describe it, but such an experience must first be felt. The student of Yoga purposely holds back from description because it is limiting; the student wants to go beyond known limits of thought. Keeping the mind empty allows increased awareness. Instead of filling the void or expanse with your own thought, with which you are already familiar, you allow new, creative, spontaneous forms to appear—forms you have never seen or experienced before. From this training, you will understand why the basis of philosophical thought in Kashmir Shaivism is called "the Yoga of delight, wonder, and astonishment." It is easy to see why people who seriously practice Yoga are never bored.

Everything a Yoga student does to lead to expansion eventually ends in transformation. Without this expansion, you can't really practice Yoga, because Yoga takes you outside your own limited fantasy of yourself while you are fully supported by the strength of yourself as an individual. This is described in Eastern poetry as a lotus resting on the water: in full bloom, yet untouched by the water.

This is also the ancient picture of *Vishnu*, asleep on the coiled serpent Kundalini, supported by the ocean of milk. The geometrical representation of this picture is the *yantra* (diagram) at the beginning of this chapter.

The "I Love You" Fantasy Technique

The "I Love You" Fantasy Technique, practiced regularly, will help to reinforce feelings of self-confidence, raise self-esteem, remove fear, and reduce the incidence of crippling "ugly fits." This technique should be done as a complement to—rather than as a substitute for—your daily meditation period as described in Chapter 2.

Start with the **Laughing Bicycle** (3.1): Lying on your back, pump your legs as if you were riding a bicycle. Pump your arms as well, and laugh out loud for several seconds. Then relax and settle into the Corpse Pose. This exercise helps to release tension and stimulates the brain chemicals that cause feelings of well-being.

Give yourself the same protections as when you are doing your regular meditation: lie on your back comfortably, without a pil-

3.1

low under your head, on your bed or the floor, or sit in a chair that keeps your back straight. Cover yourself with a blanket or shawl. Make sure your pets are in another room and turn off your telephone. Press your back slightly toward the floor, then release and relax. Pull your chin down a little toward your chest without straining, to stretch the cords in the back of the neck that will allow more movement of the feeling that will affect your brain. If your lower back is tense, place one or two pillows under your knees.

Now bring your attention to your forehead. Breathe in, saying "I love you" to yourself. Say, "I love you" as you breathe out. Repeat several times: breathe in, "I love you," and breathe out, "I love you." Now breathe in and hold for a moment. Imagine the feeling "I love you" spreading throughout your brain in a beautiful, warm, wet, perfumed essence. Breathe out, "I love you."

Now relax completely. Let your breath relax. And just hold that feeling. For a few more minutes, continue saying "I love you" as you breathe in and as you breathe out.

Now think to yourself as you breathe in and hold your breath for a moment: "Whom do I love?" Breathe out and say, "I love you." Breathe in and hold again; think: "Who loves me?" Now think to yourself: "My breath loves me." Breathe out and say, "My breath loves me." The breath is inside you. It loves you. Breathe in and think, "I'm holding my breath—it loves me." Breathe out and think, "I have released my breath—it still loves me." Take a deep breath, always through your nose. Breathe in: "My breath loves me." Breathe out: "My breath is gone now but it still loves me."

Now relax completely. Visualize the inside of your head and your body. Think of how the breath is commingled with love. Oxygen is flowing through your veins and heart and every part of you because you can't live without your breath. Visualize this loving breath inside your body. Are there any impediments keeping it from moving where it wants to go? Visualize this feeling of love and breath removing any kind of block or constriction, moving easily and sweetly throughout your body.

Bring it to your forehead. Think, "I love you—my breath is in my forehead." Relax your forehead. Now think of this feeling of love spreading to your eyes—you can almost see it! Relax your eyes and let the breath of love simply swim out into the rest of your face. Feel this breath of love in your nose, because it breathes for you. Every time you breathe in, breathe, "I love you." Every time you breathe out, breathe, "I love you." Let the breath of love flow freely so that your face melts with love. Let your mouth and throat relax, thinking, "I love you" as you breathe.

Let your neck relax now so you have no constriction that will stop the breath from moving. Love comes in with your breath—relax. Love goes out with your breath—relax. Drop your collarbone toward the floor and say, "I love you." Let the ends of your shoulders drop. Do the same with your arms; let them relax; feel that they are fully supported by this breath of love. Rest your arms in love. Relax your wrists. Let your hands be totally relaxed in love. You're vulnerable. You don't care. You can't lose love. Breath comes in and goes out, and love is still there. Relax your fingers, letting them curl slightly, like a baby's hand when it is asleep.

Now go to your chest. Be aware that you are taking a breath into your heart: "I love you." Breathe it out with love. Breathe into your lungs: "I love you." Breathe out, "I love you." Now relax your entire chest. Let your breath relax in love. Become aware that this breath is love. You're not making it happen; it's happening because it loves you.

Now breathe in and think of your stomach. Breathe out and say "I love you" as you relax your stomach. Relax your abdomen, thinking, "I love you. I love you the way you are." Now feel the breath of love move through your hip joint: warm, liquid, lubricating, beautiful—perfectly balanced and poised. Now say, "I love you" to your hips and relax them. Let the large bones in the top of your legs sink toward the floor; you don't have to hold them up. You love them. They love you. You can't lose love. Relax your legs in love. Relax your

knees and ankles and think, "I love you." Now think to your feet, "I love you." Relax your feet.

Now picture yourself just simply floating, completely supported on this breath, this love. Bring your attention up to the back of your hips and the base of your spine. Open it up like a flower. Say, "I love you." Don't fight it. Let it flow easily, smooth and quiet. Relax the back of your shoulder blades. Let your back get soft. Love is supporting you. "I love you, back." The back of your neck relaxes. Think to yourself, "I love you. I love you." Then you reach your brain, your hair, all soft and supported, resting in love, in breath.

Breathe in and think love. Breathe out—love is still there. Think of your brain floating in a pool of this love. Now make it totally quiet and say to yourself, "I love you." Bring your mind to your forehead and think nothing. Hold this feeling. If you feel any other thought coming in, make sure that it says "I love you." Transpose any thought to "I love you" and go back to thinking nothing. Think nothing as long as you can. Stop talking to yourself. Become silent internally.

Rest quietly like this for about ten minutes, then slowly stretch, take a deep breath and let it out, and think about how you feel. Rest on your side or stomach for a few minutes, enjoying the feeling before you get up. Move slowly back into your normal attitudes and lifestyle.

4
Energy

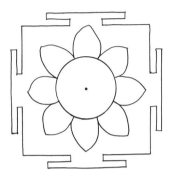

A manifestation of Surya, *the sun*

We begin with perhaps the most important sequence of movements in Yoga—the Sun Salutation, which is designed to call on the energy of the sun to bring health and vigor into the body and mind. I advise all my students to begin their daily routine with this sequence. When you do this routine, you salute the sun as the primal source of energy and ask that this energy flower in you and bring robust health. The diagram at the beginning of this chapter represents the power of the sun. If you wish, you may focus your eyes on this diagram while you do the Sun Salutation.

My teacher Rama was very specific in advising me not to practice this asan sequence while concentrating on the *setting* sun—when the sun's energy is fading into night. In fact, he advised me never to spend time *watching* the setting sun, and I never do, to this day. This sequence is only to be done while concentrating on the *rising* sun, and its light that comes powerfully into the world as you begin your day.

When Rama lived in the mountains in Kashmir, he used to do 108 repetitions of the Sun Salutation at dawn. I advise you to do no more than three. I have found that in the United States most people believe that "more is better." This is not true in the practice of Yoga asans. A person should never attempt 108 repetitions unless he or she has achieved a real mastery of Yoga.

The second sequence in this chapter, the Fatigue Routine, was developed to concentrate and conserve the energies of the body and mind. The deep relaxation and silence you will experience with this routine can help you avoid the physical and mental fatigue that often accompanies stress. Practice the Fatigue Routine when you feel especially stressed and tired, or at the end of your workday to give you a lift for the evening hours.

The Sun Salutation

The Sun Salutation stretches and strengthens all the major muscle groups in the body and exercises the respiratory system. Try to do three repetitions of the entire sequence every day once you have learned it well. To avoid strain, never practice this sequence without doing a complete warm-up routine first (see Chapter 2). If you have back or neck problems, do each movement at half capacity and do not lift your knee off the floor in Steps 4 and 10. In Steps 2 and 12, it is important to raise your arms wide to the sides to expand your chest fully before you stretch upward. This will strengthen your respiratory system and all your breathing muscles, bringing oxygen to the bottom of the lungs.

At first, as you are learning the sequence, you may have trouble breathing as directed. Practice the

sequence several times just breathing naturally until you know it well enough to add the correct breath patterns. These breath patterns are very important to the sequence, so add them as soon as possible.

At the places marked "Asan Point," try to hold the position for a few seconds with body in pose, breath held (in or out, depending on the exercise), eyes focused, and mind silent. (For more on the Asan Point, see "The Asan Point" in Chapter 1.) Hold the Asan Point only as long as it is comfortable.

To begin your routine, bring your mind and body to attention facing east, mentally visualizing the rising sun. Visualize the sun radiating throughout your body. If you wish, recite the Health Mantram (in this chapter) three times. If you do not wish to use this mantram, simply bring yourself to full attention and begin the sequence as described below.

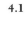

SUN SALUTATION

1. Stand with feet parallel and palms together. (This is the traditional Indian greeting of *Namasté,* or *Namaskar,* which gives the sequence its Sanskrit name: *Surya Namaskar.*) Breathe out completely (4.1).

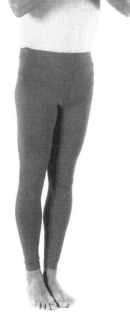

2. Breathe in as you raise your arms in a wide circle out to the sides and overhead. Stretch your arms back as you lift them to allow the fullest expansion of your chest. Press your palms together above your head and look up at your hands. Stretch up and hold your breath (4.2). *Asan Point.*

4.2

3. (a) Breathe out as you bend forward from the waist, keeping palms together, tucking your head, and keeping your back straight as long as you can (4.3). (b) When you've bent as far forward as you can comfortably, grasp the back of your

4.3

ankles, calves, or thighs (depending on limberness), bend your elbows, pull your upper body

gently toward your legs, and tuck your chin toward your chest (4.4). Hold your breath out. *Asan Point.* (Note: If you have back problems, bend forward only halfway and do not pull with your arms.)

4.4

4. Breathe in as you release your legs and stand up. Breathing out, immediately lunge forward with your right leg, keeping your toes tucked under (4.5). (Note: In subsequent repeti-

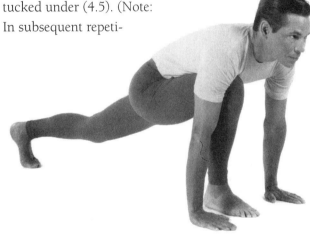

4.5

tions alternate the leg you lunge forward with; experiment to find the right distance to step forward so you can perform Steps 4 and 5 in one fluid movement. Try to keep your left knee off the floor unless you have back problems.)

5. Breathe in as you gently raise your arms in a wide circle out to the sides and overhead, palms together, looking up at your hands. Hold your breath in (4.6). *Asan Point*.

7. Hold your breath out as you lower your body so that your chin, chest, and knees touch the floor (toes are still tucked under). When your knees touch the floor, relax the held breath and start to breathe in (4.8).

8. Continue breathing in as you curl your head back, then lift your chest and stomach; your hipbones stay on the floor. (This is called the Cobra Pose.) Look up through your forehead. Hold your breath in (4.9). *Asan Point*.

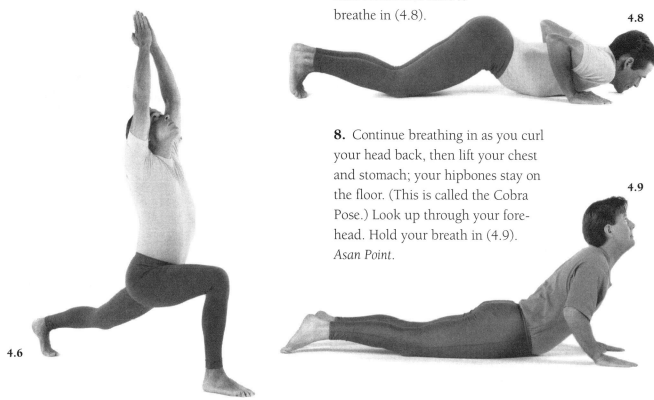

6. Breathe out, bring both hands down on the floor on either side of your right foot, bring your right foot back next to your left foot, and straighten your body into a "plank" position (4.7).

9. Breathe out as you push your hips up and heels down into a V position. Tuck your chin to your chest. Hold your breath out (4.10). *Asan Point*.

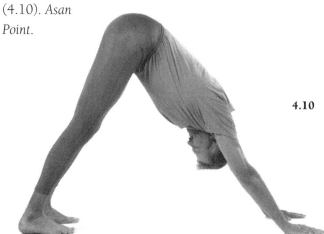

10. Start to breathe in as you bring your left foot forward between your hands and lunge forward with your left leg. Continue breathing in as you raise your arms in a wide circle to the sides and overhead, with palms together, looking up at your hands. Hold your breath in (4.11). *Asan Point*. (Note: Alternate the leg you lunge forward with in this step as you do in position 4.5. Try to keep your right knee off the floor unless you have back problems.)

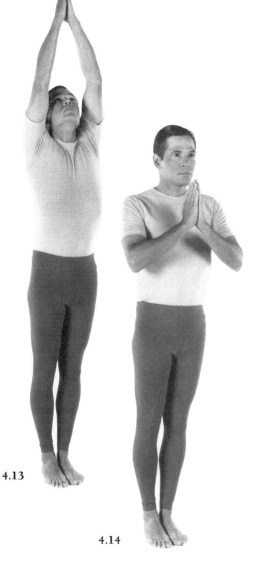

4.11

11. Breathe out as you bring your right foot forward next to the left, grasp behind your legs as in Step 3(b), tuck your chin toward your chest, and hold your breath out (4.12). *Asan Point*. (Note: If you have back problems, bend only

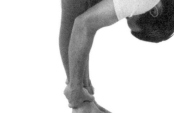

4.12

halfway down and do not pull with your arms.)

12. Breathe in as you straighten, bringing your arms in a wide circle out to the sides and overhead, palms together. Look up at your hands and stretch. Hold your breath in (4.13). *Asan Point*.

13. Breathe out as you bring your arms in a circle down to the sides and back to your chest with palms together as in Step 1 (4.14). Repeat the entire sequence three times.

4.13

4.14

A Mantram for Health

Long ago, when I was living in the jungle near Haridwar with my teacher Rama, I began using a *mantram* of the sun with my practice of the Sun Salutation. I have used it all these 40-odd years since, and have taught it to advancing students who seem capable of sincere, steady practice.

As I mentioned earlier, a *mantram* is a sound (I think of it as a mass of radiant energy) that has a particular effect on the body and mind. In Chapter 2, you read about the mantram *Om,* which is always used to precede a meditation session. Many people are curious about where and how mantrams originated—who, if anyone, first decided that this particular sound meant that particular thing? In Mantric Yoga, it is said that the relationship of a word to the object it denotes is eternal, not arbitrary, and there is a system of "natural sounds" for everything in the universe. The Sanskrit language, from which Yogic mantrams are derived, was supposedly created under this same premise, rather than evolving haphazardly over time like modern languages. The mantram to the sun that I am describing here was given to me in Sanskrit but translated by Rama into English to make it easier to remember. Rama, who had experienced the mantram in the original Sanskrit, told me the effect of the mantram would be the same for me even though I was unable to pronounce the Sanskrit correctly at that time.

Mantrams should be used only if you are a vegetarian. The body chemistry is completely different when a vegetarian diet is followed, as is the effect of mantric practice. What you eat is directly connected to the ethic of nonviolence, one of the important practices of advanced Yogic training. If you wish to use this mantram, I strongly advise you to follow my direction concerning diet.

To those who qualify and wish to use it, I give this mantram in the name of my teacher Rama, who gave it to me. First, take your concentrated position (standing, with palms together) facing east, the direction of the rising sun. It is not necessary to be outdoors, but simply to be aware of where the sun rises. (Never look at the sun directly, or you may hurt your eyes.) Remember that this mantram is to be used only while concentrating on the rising sun, so if you must schedule your practices for afternoon or evening, you should visualize the rising sun in your mind, and then begin.

First, repeat the name Rama, saluting the teacher who gave the mantram. Then proceed:

O Lord of Light, Master of Peace,
destroyer of all diseases, the Sun, I
bow down to thee, please be gracious

WHEN YOU DON'T FEEL LIKE EXERCISING . . .

Illness and languor are described in the classic Yogic texts as two of the many obstacles to concentration for the Yoga student. Many students feel guilty when these conditions arise, as if Yoga practice were expected to produce perfect health and attention instantly and perpetually. While Yoga will help you remain well, occasionally a virus or too much stress will allow some illness or lethargy to creep in.

You have probably experienced how difficult it is to keep your mind on anything when you are ill, tired, or stressed. At these times you want only to rest or escape—in sleep, or reading, or watching television. It's best not to fight these desires. Realize that the desire to escape will always be there. Try to do your daily Yoga practice during the times when you are fresh—before the most stressful part of your day—in order to keep your commitment to practicing once every twenty-four hours. Then you can let your body rest or watch television, knowing that you have kept your word to yourself and are now letting your body enjoy rest. Listen to your body and give it the rest it needs to get well and stay well. If illness is keeping you from practicing, try to do a bare minimum of Yoga practice—three minutes—and you will feel better about yourself.

Many students feel guilty when they experience languor—usually a transient state of slowness or "fogginess" of mind and body. Occasional laziness of mind is natural and to be expected—and you might be surprised to learn that it often has healing effects. Languor can be a wonderful, natural feeling. If you've already done your three minutes of exercise for the day, why not be languorous and enjoy the feeling?

unto me, O Supreme Lord or Being, and give me my desired object, the health.

Repeat this three times, then begin the Sun Salutation, trying to hold the vision of the rising sun in your mind as you practice. The combination of all these details—the sequence, mantram, and diet—will have a powerful effect in helping you reach maximum health and strength.

The Fatigue Routine

Fatigue manifests in the body and mind in several ways, most noticeably in the breath. You will find that your breath shortens as stomach muscles become rigid; you may notice yourself sighing or yawning frequently and breathing very shallowly, sometimes even holding your breath out for several seconds without realizing it. Your back tends to slump forward as your upper back and neck muscles become hot and tired; you may notice that it takes more effort to sit or stand straight. Pressure on spinal nerves and muscles from poor posture causes blood flow to the brain to be restricted; you may feel depressed, sluggish, and unable to concentrate.

The following routine helps to reenergize your body and mind by reversing these conditions through poses that compress the body forward or stretch it backward. Compression poses, such as the Baby Pose and the Spine Twist, cause you to relax your breathing muscles so you naturally breathe more deeply and completely. Compression poses also increase circulation to all parts of the body, flushing the brain, muscles, and organs with fresh oxygen. Poses that stretch the spine backward cool and shorten the postural muscles, and relieve pressure on the spinal bones and nerves. Pressure on internal organs and improved circulation cause a chemical change to take place in your body, which lifts your mood and steadies your concentration. You may feel clearer,

more alert, and happier. The Fatigue Routine is designed with minimal extraneous movement between positions so you can remain concentrated throughout the routine.

The most effective time of day to practice this routine is as soon as you get home from work. Start with a quick shower to help your mind make the transition from work to your home environment by rinsing off the tensions of the day.

At the places marked *Asan Point*, try to hold the position for a few seconds with body in pose, breath held (in or out depending on the exercise), eyes focused, and mind silent. (For more on the Asan Point, see "The Asan Point" in Chapter 1.) Hold the Asan Point only as long as it is comfortable.

This Fatigue Routine contains many rest periods in the Baby Pose because of its beneficial compression effects. If you are too stiff to rest in the Baby Pose comfortably, hold the pose for only a few seconds, then relax in the Corpse Pose.

FATIGUE ROUTINE

1. Baby Pose. Sit on your heels, rest your forehead on the floor, and let your elbows relax out to each side. Let your breath relax and rest for about one minute (4.15). (Variation: See Chapter 2 for variations on this position if you have stiff knees or hips. If you have a large midsection, keep your hips on your heels and just bend forward as far as you can.)

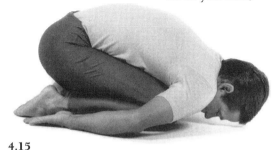

4.15

2. Pigeon Pose. (a) Slide your right leg back and place both hands on either side of your left knee. Rest your forehead on the floor (4.16). Breathe out. (b) Breathe in as you curl up, starting with your head, then your spine, looking up through your forehead the entire time (4.17). Hold your breath in. *Asan Point.*

Breathe out as you curl down, chest first, then shoulders, then head and eyes. Repeat slowly three times. (c) Push yourself up on your fists, straighten your arms, relax your back, and stare at one spot on the floor about three feet in front of you (4.18). Breathe out and hold. *Asan Point.* Breathe in as you release the position.

3. Straighten your left leg, tuck the toes under, and push your body up into a V position. Tuck your head and hold for just a moment (4.19).

4. Transition back to the **Pigeon Pose** by bending your right knee and lowering yourself into position for

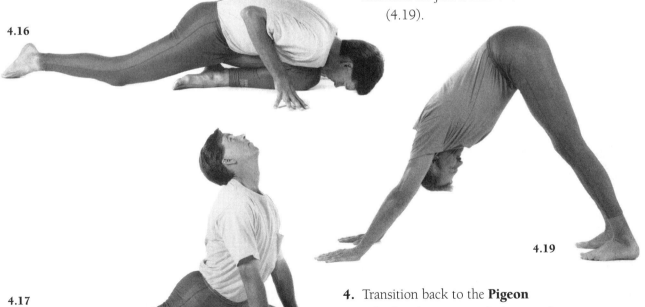

4.16

4.17

4.18

4.19

the Pigeon Pose on the other side. Repeat positions 2–4 three times.

5. Rest in the **Baby Pose** or the **Corpse Pose** until breath returns to normal (4.20).

4.20

6. Fish Pose. (a) Sit up and lean back on one elbow (4.21), then both. (b) Arch your back and gently lower yourself until the top of your head rests on the floor (4.22). Place your hands flat, palms down, at your sides. Hold for a few moments, looking up through your forehead. (c) Separate your knees and heels and gently lower

4.21

4.22

your body between your legs to lie flat (4.23) as you breathe in, then out. Hold your breath out. *Asan Point.* Breathe in as you come up out of the position. (Variation: If you are unable to do this asan with legs folded back, extend your legs straight out in front of you and point your toes. The breath pattern and Asan Point are the same.)

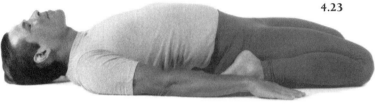

4.23

7. Rest. Push yourself up on one elbow (4.21) and come forward to rest in the Baby Pose (4.20) or the Corpse Pose.

8. Camel Pose.
(a) Come up on your knees, separate your knees slightly, arch your back, and grab your left heel with your left hand (4.24). Do this once on each side

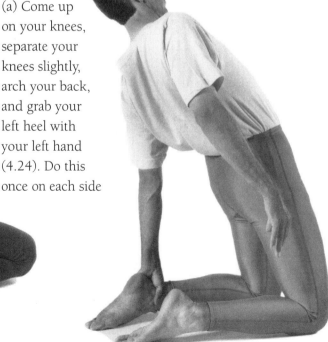

4.24

to warm up. (b) Then reach back and grab both heels (4.25). Breathe in, then let your head gently fall back as you breathe out (unless you have a disk problem in your upper back or neck, in which case keep your head up). Hold your breath out. *Asan Point.* Release and breathe in. (Variation: If you are unable to grab both heels at once, do the exercise once on each side in position 8(a) [4.24] instead.)

10. Transition to the **Hero Pose**. Place your hands on the floor in back of you and support yourself as you lift your left leg out to the side and shift your body weight so you are sitting on the floor with your right leg tucked in very close to your hip (4.27).

11. Hero Pose. (a) Lift your left foot up onto your right thigh close to your hip. The goal is to rest the top of your foot (not just the toes) on your thigh (4.28). (Variation: If your knees are stiff, just rest your left foot against the inside of your right thigh [4.29].)

9. Return to the **Baby Pose**, but this time increase the compression by making fists and placing them in your lap (4.26) so they press into your abdomen as you bend forward. Hold this position for as long as you feel comfortable.

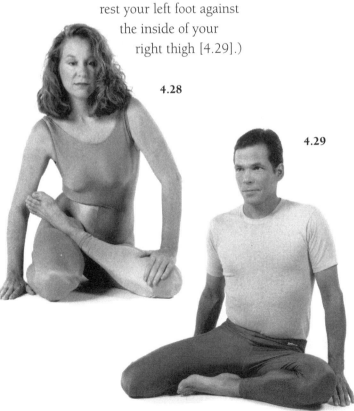

4.25

4.26

4.27

4.28

4.29

(b) Place your right hand on the outside of your right knee and apply slight pressure as you breathe in, then breathe out as you bend forward, aiming your head toward the spot just to the inside of your right knee (4.30). Hold your breath out. *Asan Point.* Breathe in and release. (Variation: If your knees and hips are quite limber, try this variation: Breathe in and come up from position 11(b), then bring your knees as close together as you can while keeping the left foot on the right thigh. Breathe in, then breathe out and bend forward, aiming your head toward the spot just *outside* your right knee. *Asan Point.* Breathe in and release.)

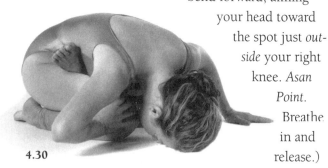

4.30

12. Hero Compression.

(a) Keeping your left foot on your right thigh, gently lift your right leg and place your right foot flat on the floor close in to your body. Your weight will shift to your left hip. With your right hand, reach around your upraised right knee and grasp the outside of the left leg. Then with your left arm, reach around your upraised right knee and grasp the right upper arm (4.31). Breathe out. Fix your gaze on one spot on the floor about three feet in front of you. Hold your breath out. *Asan Point.*

Breathe in and release. (Variation: If you are doing the Hero Pose as in position 11(a) [variation], do the compression by lifting your right leg and placing the foot flat, close to the left foot [4.32].)

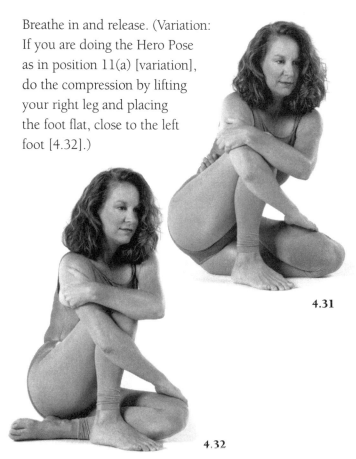

4.31

4.32

13. Transition to the **Spine Twist**.

Lower your right knee to the floor; in the same motion, grasp your left knee with your left hand and lift it up, resting your left foot on the outside of your right knee (4.33). This puts you in position for the Spine Twist.

4.33

14. Lean back on your hands and arch your back to stretch and align the vertebrae (4.34).

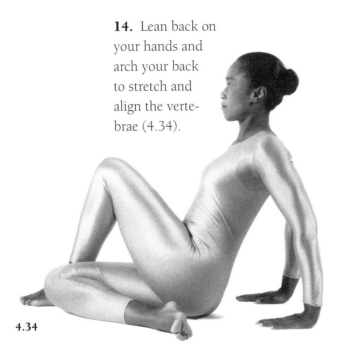

4.34

15. Spine Twist. (a) With your right arm, reach around to the *left* of your upraised left knee, push the knee to the right as far as you can, straighten your right arm, and grasp your left big toe with your right thumb and forefinger (4.35).

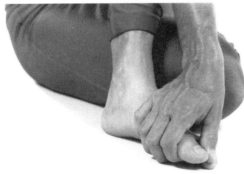

4.35

(Variation: If you cannot reach your big toe, grasp your left ankle or your right knee instead. If you cannot straighten your right arm, just bend your elbow and push back

on the knee as far as you can.)
(b) Straighten your left arm, point your fingers in toward your body, and bring your hand in close to the end of your spine. Straighten your back, look forward, breathe in, then breathe out as you twist back toward the left as far as you can (4.36). Fix your gaze on one spot slightly above eye level. Hold your breath out. *Asan Point.*

4.36

(Variation: If you have knee problems, try this easier version of the **Spine Twist**: keep your right leg straight [4.37].) (c) Relax your breath, turn your head forward, release your right hand, and turn it back to grasp the heel of your right foot. Place your left hand a little further to the back, straighten

4.37

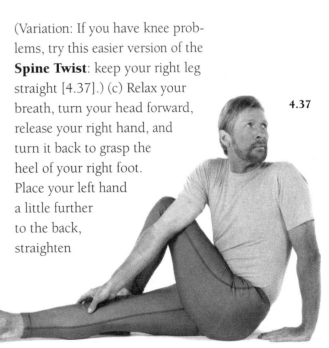

your arm and your back, breathe in again, then breathe out and turn to the left again, as far as you can (4.38). Fix your eyes on one spot slightly above eye level. Hold your

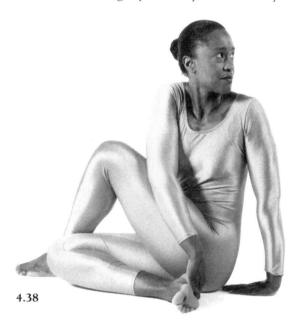

4.38

breath out. *Asan Point.* Breathe in and release. (d) Turn back to face forward, slide your left foot back, and let your knee drop slightly. Bend forward, aiming your head between

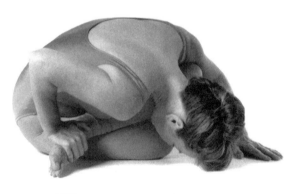

4.39

your right knee and left foot (4.39). Hold for a few seconds.

16. Transition to opposite side. Straighten up, grasp your left heel with your left hand and lift it up, around, and back so it rests next to your left hip. Lift your right foot onto your left thigh (4.40). You are now ready to repeat positions 11–15 (Hero Pose, Hero Compression, and Spine Twist) on the opposite side.

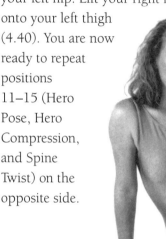

4.40

17. Transition to the **Diamond Pose**. After completing position 15 on the opposite side, grasp your right foot with your right hand and place it sole to sole with your left foot.

18. Diamond Pose. Lace your fingers around your toes, straighten your back, breathe in (4.41), then

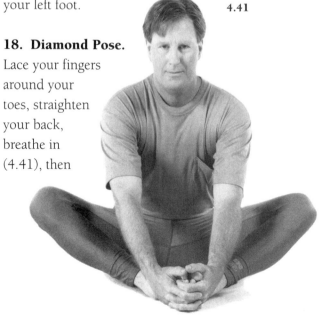

4.41

breathe out and bend forward as far as you can without strain (4.42). Hold your breath out.

Asan Point. Breathe in and release.

19. Rest on your back in the Corpse Pose for at least one minute (4.43).

Finish the routine with at least five minutes of Complete Breath and twenty to thirty minutes of meditation in a lying down position (unless you are *extremely* comfortable in a seated position).

4.42

4.43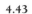

5
Strength

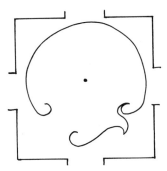

*Ganesh, energy, the product of union of the male/female
principles; a symbol of strength, wisdom, and success*

The concept of strength has many aspects in Yoga. On the physical level, strengthening and toning of the muscles, joints, and connective tissues contributes to a healthier body, with better posture, greater resistance to illness, more stamina, and a stronger cardiovascular system. Many of the asans in the Strength Routine will also help to strengthen your bones because they are *weight-bearing* exercises—that is, they ask you to partially support your weight on your hands, shoulders, or other joints, which builds bone tissue when done regularly.

Many students who begin to practice Yoga mistakenly believe that limberness is the primary goal. Limberness is an important objective in Hatha Yoga, contributing to a more comfortable seated position and more relaxed muscles and joints, but if you do not also strengthen the joints, they may become weak and more susceptible to injury. Many people emphasize either strength *or* limberness. Strength *with* limberness is the special contribution of Yoga. The combination of limberness and strength is one of the many approaches that lead to unrestricted enjoyment. Unrestricted enjoyment is beauty, and beauty is a quality of Yoga.

On a more subtle level, Yoga strengthens the will. People who lack decisiveness will benefit from practicing strengthening exercises on a regular basis. If you find it difficult to practice every day after you have told yourself that you will do so, you can suspect a weak will. This routine will help strengthen your will so you can more easily follow through with what you want to do. Willpower is directly related to truthfulness, one of the ten ethical observances that are followed by serious Yoga practitioners (see Chapter 6). Observing your ability to do what you say you are going to do will give you great insight into your practice of truthfulness. Keeping your word, even casually, is a dramatic achievement in the strengthening of your will. The old books say that when you become established in truthfulness, your words become very powerful because what you say becomes true; this only happens with a strong will. You can see that if you were consciously practicing this discipline, you would learn to be very careful of everything you said, even in jest.

GANESH: A SYMBOL FOR STRENGTH

The diagram at the beginning of this chapter is a representation of the elephant-headed god Ganesh who, in mythology, is the son of Shiva (the male principle) and Parvati (the female principle). Ganesh represents energy, the principle of strength, and the overcoming of obstacles, as an elephant forges ahead through the jungle without any difficulty. He is also recognized as the force of wisdom and success. If you wish, you may use the dot in the center of the diagram as a focusing point during your asan routine.

The following qualities are surely always found in the bodies of every Yogi: strong appetite, good digestion, cheerfulness, handsome figure, great courage, mighty enthusiasm, and full strength.

(Siva Samhita)

In this chapter you will learn the Strength Routine, a very demanding sequence of Yoga exercises that strengthens the muscles, nerves, connective tissue, and joints, as well as improving mental strength. Medical research has found that even thinking about raising your arm increases blood flow to the arm and the brain centers responsible for that action. The Strength Routine calls for great mental attention along with physical exertion. In order to build strength in the muscle fibers, the muscle must be contracted to at least 75 percent of its capacity. Most of the positions in this routine fulfill this requirement. If you are unable at first to practice the entire routine as instructed without tiring to the point of exhaustion, start with fewer repetitions and more rests between exercises: in other words, go for quality rather than quantity.

Be sure you are breathing correctly in each position in order to increase oxygen flow to the muscles and avoid buildup of carbon dioxide and other waste products that are given off when a muscle is exercised, and can result in stiffness or pain. Many of the poses call for a natural breath, which will probably be somewhat faster than your normal breath, due to the exertion. Hold your breath only during the Asan Point. Always breathe through your nose, and focus on the steamlike sound of the breath. You will multiply the beneficial effects of the routine by practicing the sequence with your full attention, both in the transitions between poses and in the Asan Point. The Strength Routine is somewhat longer than the other routines in this book; it may take thirty to forty minutes. This routine should be done slowly and deliberately—never quickly.

At the places marked *Asan Point*, try to hold the position for a few seconds with body in pose, breath held (in or out, depending on the exercise), eyes focused, and mind silent. (For more on the Asan Point, see "The Asan Point" in Chapter 1.) Hold the Asan Point only as long as it is comfortable.

The Strength Routine

1. Hip Rotation. Stand with hands on lower back: spread fingers to support lower back and hook thumbs over hips. Separate feet as far as you can comfortably, and point your toes forward. Keep your legs straight but

do not lock your knees (5.1). Rotate hips five times in each direction. Breathe naturally.

2. Windmill. Keep your hands and feet as they were in Step 1. Knees should remain straight but not locked throughout the movement. Breathe in and swivel toward the right, then breathe out as you bend your head toward your right knee (5.2) and across to your left knee. Start to breathe in as you lift up to a standing position (facing left) and swivel to the right to begin your second repetition. Repeat three to six times to the right, then three to six times to the left.

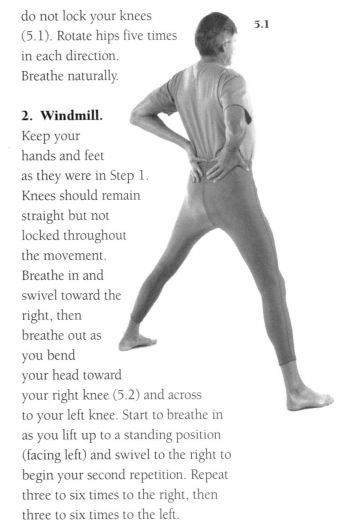

5.1

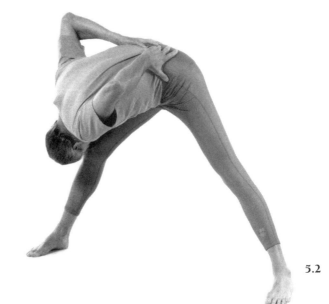

5.2

3. Triangle Series. (a) With feet in same position as Step 2, breathe in, then breathe out as you bend forward and place both hands on the floor in front of your feet (5.3). Stretch and hold your breath out. *Asan Point.* (b) Breathe in and release, then breathe out as you grasp both ankles, pull gently, and hold your breath out (5.4).

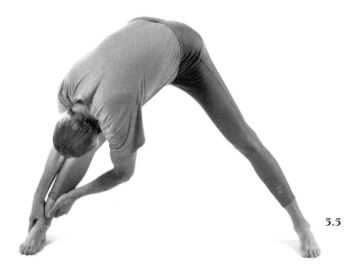

5.5

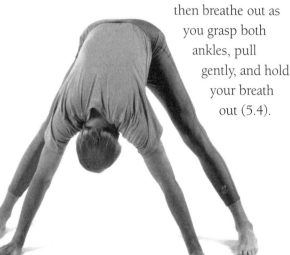

5.3

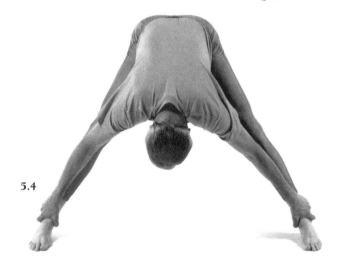

5.4

and repeat with the left ankle, holding your breath out as you pull toward the left leg. *Asan Point.* (d) Breathe in and release, then while keeping your heels on the floor, toes pointed slightly inward, walk your hands out in front of you as far as you can, then bend your elbows and stretch your head toward the floor (5.6). Hold for a moment. (e) Come up slightly and walk both hands over toward the left. Bend

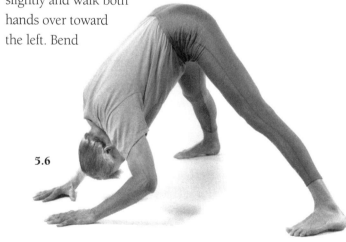

5.6

Asan Point. (c) Breathe in and release, then breathe out as you reach over to hold your right ankle with both hands, pull gently, and hold your breath out (5.5). *Asan Point.* Breathe in

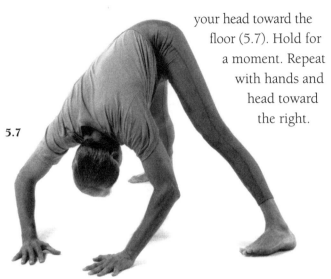

5.7

your head toward the floor (5.7). Hold for a moment. Repeat with hands and head toward the right.

4. Lunge Stretch. Breathe in as you turn completely toward the left and bend your left leg, bringing your left elbow underneath your left knee and resting on both fists (5.8). Keep your right leg straight if you can; if that position is too strenuous, rest your knee on the floor. Bend your head toward the floor as you breathe out. Hold your breath out. *Asan Point.* Breathe in and release. Repeat on the right side with the right leg.

5. Lunge Series. (a) Breathe in as you turn back to the left. Breathe out as you rest both elbows on the floor with your left elbow inside your left knee, lower your right knee to the floor, clasp your hands, and bend your head toward your hands (5.9).

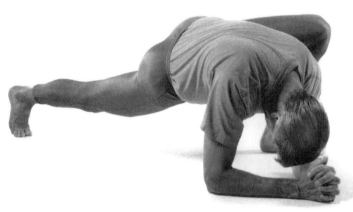

5.9

Hold your breath out. *Asan Point.*
(b) Breathe in as you push yourself up, rest your left arm on your left thigh, and straighten your right arm and your right leg (5.10). Breathe out and hold your breath out. *Asan Point.*

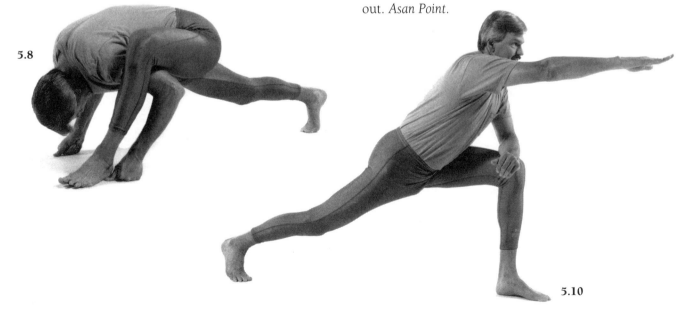

5.8

5.10

(c) Breathe in and release. With your legs in the same position, breathe out as you stretch both arms out to the sides, resting your chest on your left thigh (5.11). Hold your breath out. *Asan Point.*

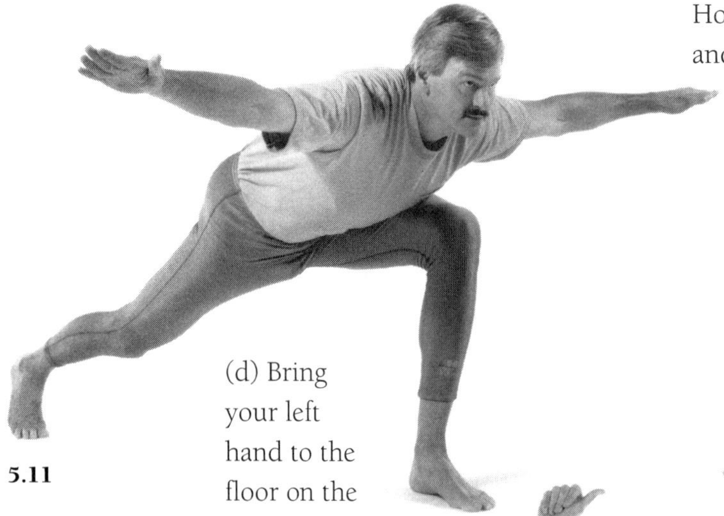

6. Bring both hands together on the floor and bring your right foot back to join your left foot. Breathe out as you press up into a V position, tucking your head and pressing your heels toward the floor (5.13). Hold for a moment. Breathe in and release.

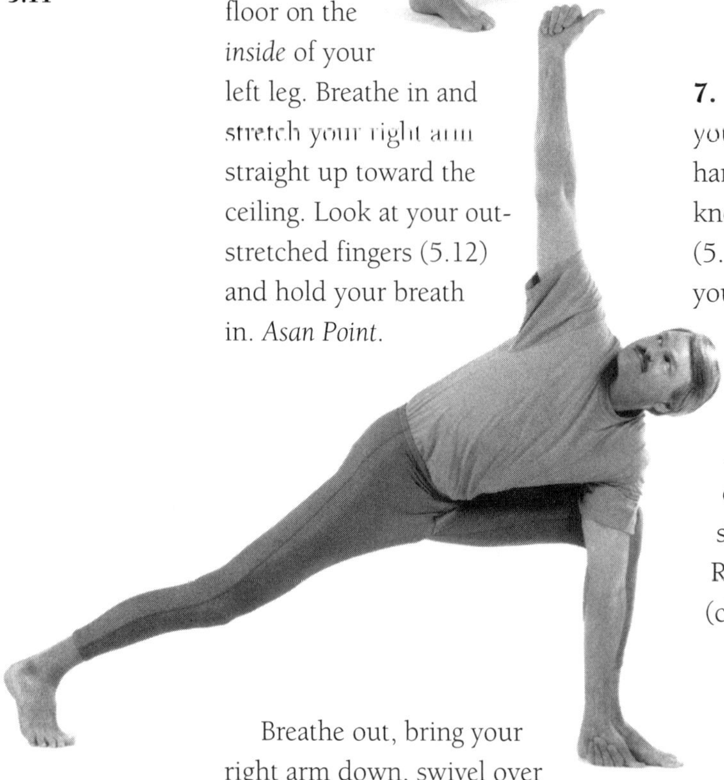

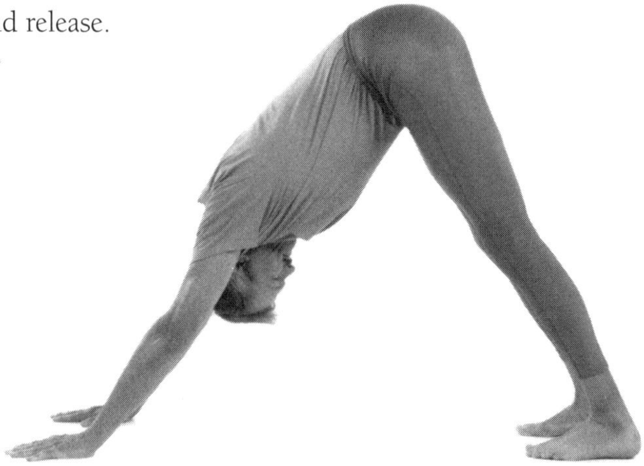

(d) Bring your left hand to the floor on the *inside* of your left leg. Breathe in and stretch your right arm straight up toward the ceiling. Look at your outstretched fingers (5.12) and hold your breath in. *Asan Point.*

5.11

5.13

7. Pigeon Pose and Hold. (a) Slide your right leg back and place both hands on either side of your left knee. Rest your forehead on the floor (5.14). Breathe out. (b) Breathe in as you curl up, starting with your head, then your spine, looking up through your forehead the entire time (5.15). Hold your breath in. *Asan Point.* Breathe out as you curl down again: chest first, then shoulders, then head and eyes. Repeat slowly three times. (c) Return to the starting

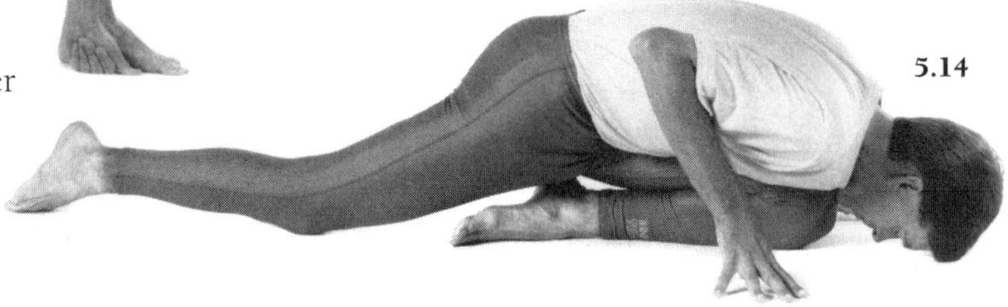

Breathe out, bring your right arm down, swivel over to the right, and repeat Step 5 on your right side.

5.12

5.14

position (5.14). Lace your fingers together in back, trying to press your palms together. If you can, straighten your elbows to squeeze your shoulder blades together—your arms will then stretch away from your body (5.16). (d) Holding that position, breathe in as you curl up and back, using your back muscles and looking up through your forehead (5.17).

5.15

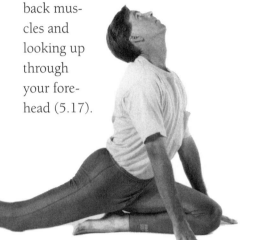

5.16

Hold your breath in. *Asan Point.* Breathe out and curl down, chest first, then head. Repeat three times. (e) Push yourself up on your fists, straighten your arms, relax your back, and stare at one spot on the floor about three feet in front of you (5.18). Breathe out and hold your breath out. *Asan Point.* Breathe in and release.

Push up just enough to slide your left leg back and right leg forward and repeat Step 7 on your right side.

5.17

Transition to the **Back Strengthener Series**. From the last holding position, release and push up, sliding your right leg back. Lower yourself to the floor on your stomach and rest, arms at your sides and head turned to one side.

5.18

8. Back Strengthener Series.
(a) Stretch your arms on the floor over your head and place your forehead on the floor. Breathe out. Breathe in as you lift arms, legs, and head, looking up through your forehead (5.19). This position is called the **Boat Pose**. Hold your

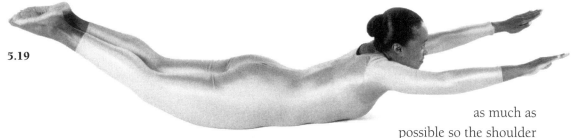

5.19

breath in. *Asan Point.* (b) Breathe out and release, bringing both arms straight out to the sides, palms down, and forehead to the floor. Rest a moment, then breathe in as you lift arms, legs, and head, looking up through your forehead (5.20). Hold your breath in. *Asan Point.* (c) Breathe out and release,

as much as possible so the shoulder blades are squeezed together and arms stretch away from the body (5.22). Look up through your forehead. Hold your breath in. *Asan Point.* (e) Breathe out and release, bending your knees and grasping your feet with both hands. Rest a moment with forehead to floor, then breathe in as you lift, pulling up on your feet so you balance on your stomach (5.23). This position is also called the **Bow Pose.** Look up through your forehead. Hold your breath in. *Asan Point.* Breathe out and

5.20

bringing your arms down to your sides. Rest a moment, then breathe in as you lift arms, legs, and head, looking up through your forehead (5.21). Hold your breath in. *Asan Point.* (d) Breathe out and release, bringing your arms behind your back with fingers clasped. Rest a moment, then breathe in as you lift arms, legs, and head, pressing your palms together and straightening your arms

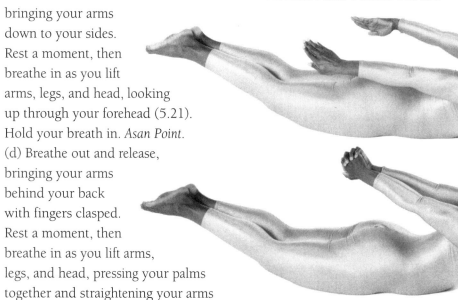

5.21

5.22

5.23

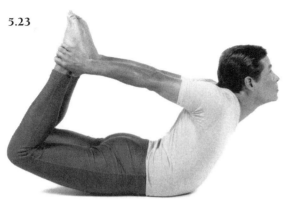

Asan Point. (b) Breathe in as you lower your body into a modified Cobra position, keeping arms and legs straight with only hands and feet touching the floor. Look up toward the ceiling (5.25). Hold your breath in. *Asan Point.* Repeat three to six times.

release, and rest on your stomach. (Variation: For an even more challenging sequence, repeat Step 8 three times: once in order from [a] to [e], then starting at [e] and moving back to [a], then forward again.)

9. Cobra V-Raise. (a) Breathe in as you push up on your hands and feet into a V position, tucking your head and pushing your heels toward the floor (5.24). Breathe out and hold your breath out.

5.25

10. Cobra V-Raise Variation. Do one to three additional repetitions of the Cobra V-Raise, but in the V position raise one leg straight (5.26). Do the same number of repetitions on each side, alternating legs.

5.24

5.26

11. From the last V position, walk your hands back toward your feet, stretch your head toward your knees, breathe out completely, and hold the breath out (5.27). *Asan Point.* Breathe in and release.

13. T Pose. Clasp your hands loosely in back and rest them on your hips. Breathe out as you lean forward and balance on your right leg, lifting your left leg parallel to the floor. Your head, neck, and the lifted leg should be in a straight line (5.29). Look at one spot on the floor. Hold your breath out. *Asan Point.* (Note: To check your position from time to time, practice in front of a mirror; hold on to a chair back or other support for balance [5.30].)

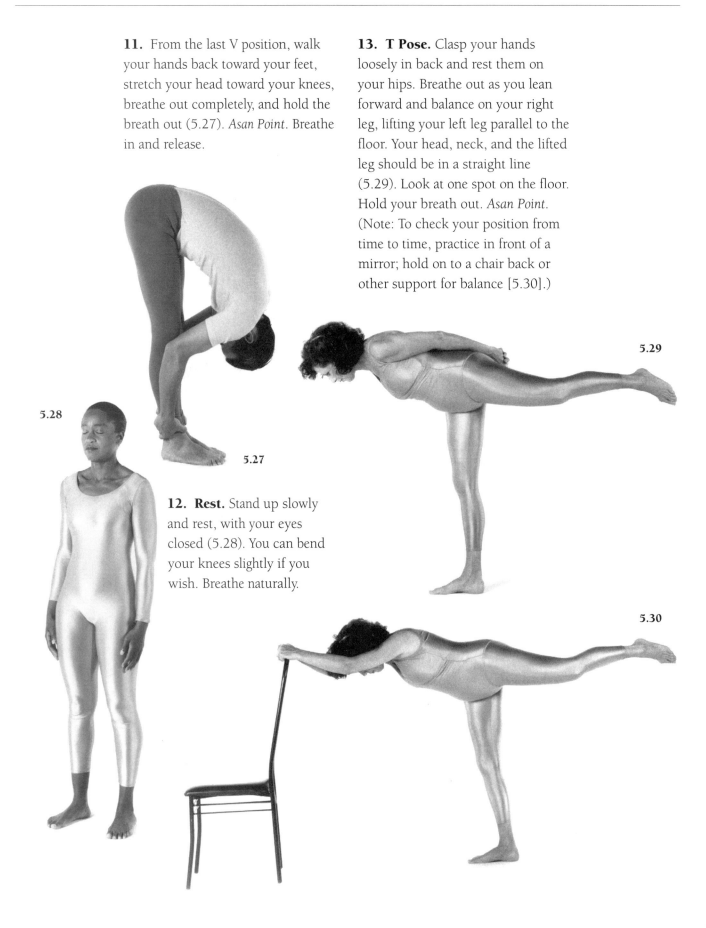

5.28

5.27

5.29

12. Rest. Stand up slowly and rest, with your eyes closed (5.28). You can bend your knees slightly if you wish. Breathe naturally.

5.30

14. T Pose Knee Bends. Release your breath and breathe naturally. Keeping your torso and lifted leg straight and parallel to the floor, gently bend your right (supporting) knee and straighten, up to three times (5.31). Try to do this without letting your shoulders and

5.31

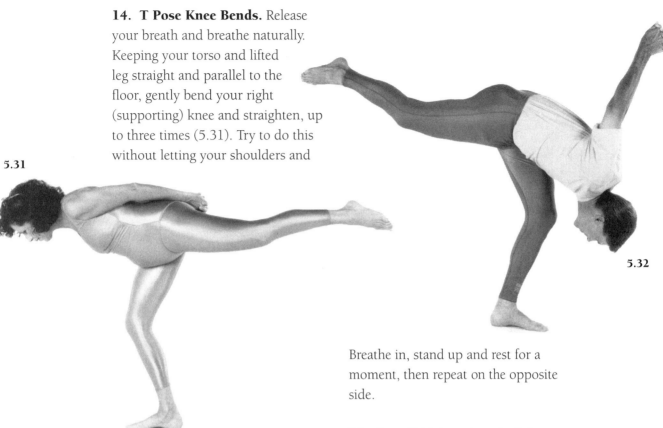

5.32

head bend toward the floor while your knee is bent. Keep breathing naturally. After the last bend, stand up and rest, then repeat Steps 13 and 14 on the opposite side.

15. Warrior Pose Variation. Straighten your arms in back so your shoulder blades are squeezed together and arms come away from your body. Breathe in. Breathe out as you bend your left knee and rest your chest on your thigh. Lift your right leg as high as possible and keep it straight (5.32). Stare at one spot on the floor. Hold your breath out. *Asan Point.*

Breathe in, stand up and rest for a moment, then repeat on the opposite side.

16. Rest. Fold down into the Baby Pose (5.33) and rest until breath returns to normal (at least one minute). Remember to try to keep your hips resting on your heels.

17. Big Sit-Up. (a) Sit up and carefully stretch both legs to the front, then lie on your back, arms overhead (5.34). Breathe out. (b) Breathe in as you lift arms and legs and try to touch your

5.33

5.34

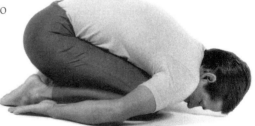

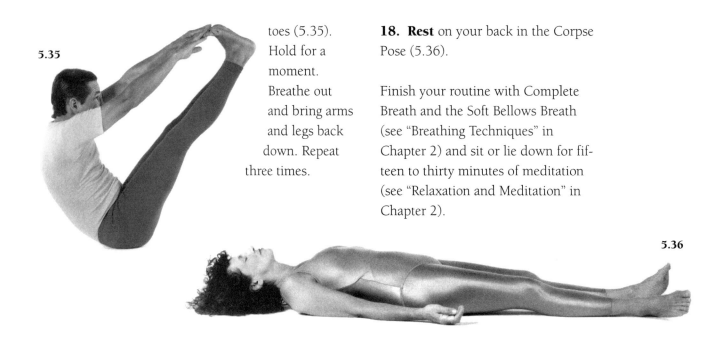

5.35

toes (5.35). Hold for a moment. Breathe out and bring arms and legs back down. Repeat three times.

18. Rest on your back in the Corpse Pose (5.36).

Finish your routine with Complete Breath and the Soft Bellows Breath (see "Breathing Techniques" in Chapter 2) and sit or lie down for fifteen to thirty minutes of meditation (see "Relaxation and Meditation" in Chapter 2).

5.36

AEROBICS AND YOGA

Fitness-oriented students often try to practice a variety of types of exercise, including aerobic exercise, in which the heart rate is raised to a "target zone" for a specified period of time. While there is nothing wrong with this, there is no need to add aerobic exercise to your practice of Yoga. If you wish to do some extra aerobic exercise a few times a week, this will not conflict with Yoga practice, but it should be done for your own enjoyment, separately from your Yoga routine.

I feel compelled in this chapter on strength to comment on the special heart-strengthening abilities of Yoga, as taught to me by my teachers. In the forty-plus years that I have been teaching, I have used this information with my students with great success.

According to my teachers, Yoga exercise and meditation allow the body to set its own correct heart rate without relying on artificial numbers determined by a general formula. In Yoga, formulas have no meaning because each person is different. Daily practice of Yoga asans helps the heart reach and maintain this optimum level of conditioning. Simultaneously, Yoga meditation brings out the subtle quality of balance in all the body's physical and chemical systems.

Yoga begins with the principle that each person has an inborn, unique pattern of heart conditioning that can be brought to maximum strength and health simply by practicing Yoga asans daily. As few as three Yoga exercises a day, done regularly and absolutely correctly, along with daily meditation, can help bring all the body's systems into balance.

Yoga benefits the cardiovascular system in other ways as well. The precise stretching and compression movements work on blood vessels as well as muscle and connective tissue, increasing their flexibility and resilience, and keeping them free-flowing. The breathing and meditation techniques, practiced daily, help to relax all the muscles and nerves, including the fine muscles that can constrict blood vessels.

Asans were invented to keep practitioners completely healthy in a very small space—a cave or a small room—where they could live and practice in seclusion. Most of the asans were designed to imitate different animals and identify with the beautiful, subtle qualities of those beings. When asans, breathing techniques, and meditation are practiced together, the result is increased strength, health, and optimum well-being.

6
Flexibility

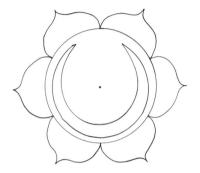

One representation of the element water

The diagram above is a representation of the element water. Water has many meanings in legend and myth; in a dream, for instance, moving through a body of water often signifies a change of consciousness. Water has no shape of its own. It seems to have no strength, yet it can wear down rock over time. Water is constantly changing: ocean tides are pulled by the moon, rivers rise and fall with the seasons, the color of water changes depending on what is suspended in or reflected in it.

Once when I was in Kashmir with Lakshmanjoo, we were riding across the lake in a small boat. I asked him why Yogis love water so much. He said, "Because it has no resistance." In Yoga the qualities of water are often imitated. Like water, a Yogi strives to be able to change course "on a dime," ready for any new experience or thought beyond what is expected or imagined. I often counsel my students to wake up in the morning and say, "Today is a good day to lose!" Everyone makes plans, and most people become extremely upset when their plans are foiled. Water has no resistance to changing its course; it takes the shape of whatever container it is put in. You will enjoy life and Yoga practice much more if you try to practice adjusting to unexpected changes more readily. Make it a game: in the morning, make your plans for the day, and watch how you feel if the day does not progress as you expected.

Try bringing the idea of fluidity into your practice of Yoga. Imagine your body taking on the flowing, beautiful quality of water as you move from one exercise to another, or even from one thought to another. Flexibility of mind and body is one of the beauties of age. When students achieve the silken movement that means there is no painful resistance in the body and the mind, they appear youthful and their faces become radiant. The years may show, but people who have this flexible quality look beautiful and appealing. You want to be near them. Flexibility is not only a physical gift, but an aura that surrounds and comforts you, no matter what your condition or age.

Flexibility in Thought: Tapas

Tapas (tolerance) is one of the ten ethical guidelines (called *yamas* and *niyamas*, meaning *restraints* and *observances*, respectively) that are vital for the practice of Yoga; the others are *ahimsa* (nonviolence), *satya* (truthfulness), *asteya* (refraining from stealing), *brahmacharya* (refraining from casual sex), *aparigrapha* (not hoarding), *saucha* (cleanliness), *santosha* (contentment), *svadyaya* (study), and *ishwara pranidhana* (remembrance). Whenever I use the word *ethics* in this book, I am referring to these ten guidelines that all serious Yoga students follow. Note that the term refers to observances as well as restraints; most people associate the concept of ethics only with prohibitions. A much wider viewpoint is used in Yoga, one that includes qualities such as contentment, purity, study, tolerance, and remembrance. I consider these ethical observances, and they are very important in Yoga.

The word *tapas* is usually translated as asceticism, austerity, self-study, and resignation. This certainly sounds like an unfriendly beginning to Yoga, because all of these terms, for most people, imply hardship or suffering, and many people believe that suffering and pain are necessary for spiritual growth or even physical fitness (as in the popular phrase "No pain, no gain").

The meaning of these terms in Yoga dialogue is entirely different. Yoga is done only for yourself, not for any other person or organization. Yoga practice needs to be approached as a friendly interplay between body and mind that helps one become healthy and strong, rather than as a harsh, forceful discipline. True Yoga practice never causes suffering or pain. In fact, students are encouraged to choose qualities of the path that will be most easy and enjoyable. Your whole Yoga practice then becomes a delight. One of the cardinal rules in Yoga is nonviolence—beginning with nonviolence toward yourself. As a Yoga student, you try never to cause yourself pain. You are not your enemy; you are your friend. In Yoga practice, tapas and the other ethical observances provide a protective atmosphere for students that keeps them from being harmed by stress.

How does Yogic philosophy define tapas, then? In my long conversations with Lakshmanjoo, we discussed each of the ten ethical guidelines in great detail. When Lakshmanjoo talked about tapas, he used the word *tolerance*, meaning "How much can you stand?" It is important to note that he is talking about how much you can stand *happily*—not in pain or suffering. Yoga is not a harsh endurance test. Every person differs in the amount of tolerance he or she can call on at first, but tolerance grows with practice; the stronger you get, the more you can take.

In Yoga, the greatest austerity a student can practice is constant attention to this code of ethics. Nonethical behavior—revenge, selfishness, lying, stealing, promiscuity, and so on—has been called life's greatest indulgence and one of its dearest pleasures. Training oneself away from this indulgence is extremely difficult—but absolutely essential for progress in Yoga. Many people blame outside forces for what they do ("The devil made me do it"). A Yogi would say, "I have a choice, and the responsibility for that action is entirely my own."

According to Lakshmanjoo, the practice of real tapas causes an internal transformation that would show outwardly as a constant change in behavior; this appears as a greater evenness and steadiness, and although upsets still occur, their results are not so devastating. Any action (provided it does not cause violence to anyone or anything) can be used to practice tapas; it is not limited to your daily Yoga routines. You have to live it. It is not something separate from yourself, your work, or your family.

This sounds like a simple task, but in the end you realize, with great humility, how difficult it really is. I used to shell peas and pack them in quart jars, a task that I chose because it was monotonous and tiresome. As I did it, I tried to transform my outlook about it so I could endure it with happiness. It taught me patience.

To practice tapas correctly you must inspect all words and actions to see if they conform to the ten qualities in Yoga's ethical framework, and that is a lot of hard work. It is putting the yoke on yourself and submitting to it with happy resignation, because the gifts gained for yourself are far more valuable than the "freedom" of indulgence. People who continually go for indulgence are never contented; in fact, they often seem trapped by their impulses, careening from one to the next like the ball in a pinball machine.

In the Introduction I stated that Yoga training allows you to add the equivalent of a second whole person to yourself in strength and creativity. This is sometimes a difficult process, because most people think of their inner and outer personas as separate. As a way to better understand tapas and the importance of this and other ethical observances, you might look at it as if you were playing the ultimate game; that is, you are playing yourself as an opponent, cajoling yourself to join yourself in play; testing yourself, pushing yourself to compete and win, experiencing both victory and defeat, gradually joining your inner self to your outer self. It is a secret game. These are self-victories that you talk about only to yourself.

You can actually picture yourself as two people: one operating in the heart and head, and the other in the outer body. In this game you yourself are the ultimate opponent. How fascinating it is to play yourself! Each opponent knows everything about the other, and they can play the game any time they like. Both participants are always available to play; both sides are very aware when victory goes to one or the other. If you fail to keep your word, for instance, both people in you are perfectly aware of it. Seeing this as a game has the delightful quality of showing you daily the relative strengths and weaknesses of both parties and the choices each one makes. This game strengthens willpower, and, as the

years go by, any little victory should be much celebrated and rewarded.

The final result of this training is that you become an extremely observant and powerful person—the sum total of two points of view, with a choice in every action you take. The ethical observances of your training become both the source of your strength and your protection. For instance, keeping your word makes your willpower very strong, and it protects you from the destructive consequences of lying.

There are some psychological theories that say we need to reexperience old, painful, emotional injuries in order to be free from them. In Yoga, this is not so. The old injuries can be worked out of the mind and body easily when they are supported totally by Yogic discipline. This purifying practice then becomes happy and comfortable. The *Hatha Yoga Pradipika* says:

Hatha Yoga is a refuge for those who are scorched by the three fires: the fire of self-created suffering, the fire of suffering through higher powers, and the fire of suffering caused by other beings.

As a teacher, I have noticed that when my students experience sadness or upset, it is always because they have moved away from the support of the ten ethical guidelines listed earlier. Ethics is always the most comforting, happy part of practices. If you can examine all actions through the filter of this ethical code, and then enjoy them, you have reached tapas.

When I first went to India to live in the jungle with my teacher Rama, I once heard wild elephants on the islands in the Ganges crying at night. Rama explained that one of them had been captured and the herd was crying out for him. The capture of these wild elephants is dangerous work, and if someone is lucky enough to be successful in it, the care and training of the animal becomes a lifelong partnership, very much like being married to a huge Caterpillar tractor—although the elephant has responses and feelings!

The young elephant is trained by being yoked between two huge domesticated buffaloes, each of which weighs over a thousand pounds, so that he is forced to move with them at every turn. You can see that the elephant's movements would be somewhat subdued! The trainer becomes the elephant's constant companion: they live, eat, and sleep together; the trainer bathes the elephant, sings to him, and speaks to him adoringly. After some time, the elephant begins to conform to the desires of the trainer; eventually he moves mountains for him. Throughout this lifelong partnership, the trainer and elephant develop tremendous respect for each other.

Most of you are so clever that you have already figured out the resemblance of this story to ourselves. A powerful resource lies within us, weighed down in the harness of physical limitation. We sense this enormous power within ourselves, but are unable to break free to use it. This is a perfect picture of the human condition: we are limited by the body, yet all the time we feel the ecstatic pull of the unbridled mind, with its ability to soar and create in wild, free expansion. Yogic philosophy says that these two seemingly separate states can become one tremendously powerful unit; all training leads to that end, at which time separateness is lost. Yoga means "yoke"; if approached properly, it is the bridge that joins the physical and mystical qualities of a person together.

The Flexibility Routine

The Flexibility Routine includes exercises to stretch and limber the major muscle groups in the spine, back of the legs, and hip and knee joints. The routine includes several challenging exercises, including a few asans practiced in the Lotus Position. The Lotus Pose requires not only extremely limber knees and hips but a very strong back. You should not try the Lotus or any of the Lotus asans if you have any trouble with your lower back.

If your knees and hips are extremely stiff, the best way to

loosen them is to sit cross-legged as often as you can throughout the day. Massaging the joints also helps, especially before and after exercises such as the Hero Poses. Never bounce or jerk in any of the positions; the best stretch comes from a comfortable holding position with the body and mind relaxed, focused, and quiet. Pay attention to the Asan Point in each exercise. If you feel soreness in your muscles the next day, you've stretched too far. Try taking a warm shower or bath before exercising to increase muscle looseness as well as to relax your entire body and mind.

At the places marked *Asan Point*, try to hold the position for a few seconds with the body in pose, breath held (in or out, depending on the exercise), eyes focused, and mind silent. (For more on the Asan Point, see "The Asan Point" in Chapter 1.) Hold the Asan Point only as long as it is comfortable.

1. Standing Sun Pose.
(a) Stand with feet together. Keep your knees straight but not locked. Breathe out. Breathe in as you raise your arms in a wide circle out to the sides and overhead. Stretch and look up at your hands (6.1). Hold your breath in. *Asan Point*. (b) Breathe out as you bend forward from the waist, keeping your hands

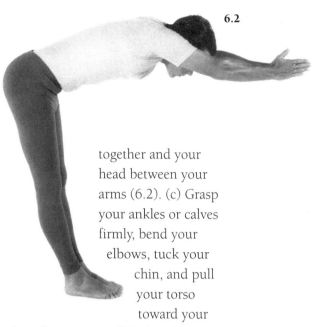

6.2

together and your head between your arms (6.2). (c) Grasp your ankles or calves firmly, bend your elbows, tuck your chin, and pull your torso toward your legs (be sure to pull by bending your elbows instead of straining your lower back). Keep your knees straight and hold your breath out (6.3). *Asan Point*. (Note: If you have back or neck problems, bend only halfway down, and do not pull your torso in.) (d) Release and breathe in as you slowly straighten, bringing your arms in a wide circle to the sides and over your head. Look up and stretch as in 1(a). Hold your breath in. *Asan Point*. Breathe out and slowly lower your arms to your sides. Repeat three times.

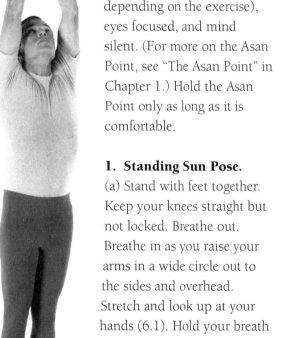

6.1

6.3

2. Triangle Poses. (a) **Alternate Triangle.** Separate your feet and point your toes inward. Breathe in and stretch your arms out to the sides (6.4), then breathe out as you bend toward

6.4

your right leg. Remember to keep your knees straight but not locked. Holding your breath out, grasp the ankle firmly with both hands, bend your elbows, and pull gently, keeping your knees straight and tucking your chin into your chest (6.5).

6.5

Hold your breath out. *Asan Point.* Breathe in as you return to the starting position. Repeat three times to each leg, alternating. (b) **Side Triangle.** From the starting position, breathe in completely, arms outstretched, then breathe out and bend sideways toward the right, sliding your right hand down your right leg. Bring your left arm up and over your head, keeping it as straight as possible; stretch from your waist. Look at a spot on the wall straight in front of you (6.6). Hold your breath out. *Asan Point.*

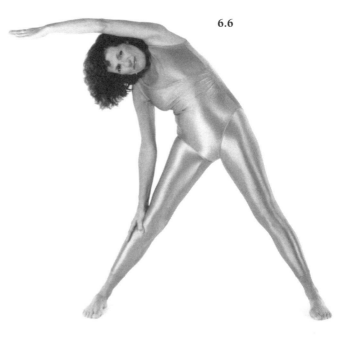

6.6

Breathe in as you return to the starting position. Repeat three times to each side, alternating. (c) **Twisting Triangle.** From the starting position, breathe in completely, arms outstretched, then breathe out as you bend toward your left leg. Grasp the *outside* of your left leg with your right hand and pull gently as you twist your torso left, bring your left arm straight up toward the ceiling. Make a loose fist with your upraised hand and look at your left thumb (6.7). Hold your breath out. *Asan Point.* Breathe in as you return to your starting position. Repeat three times on each side, alternating.

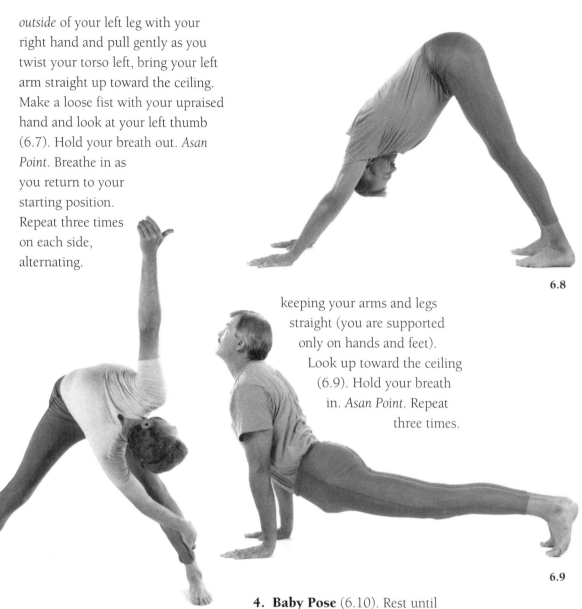

6.8

keeping your arms and legs straight (you are supported only on hands and feet). Look up toward the ceiling (6.9). Hold your breath in. *Asan Point.* Repeat three times.

6.9

6.7

3. Cobra V-Raise. Bring your feet together, bend forward, and walk your hands out to the V position (6.8). Tuck your head, push your heels to the floor, and breathe out. Hold your breath out. *Asan Point.* Breathe in as you lower your hips toward the floor and arch your back,

4. Baby Pose (6.10). Rest until breath returns to normal, at least one minute.

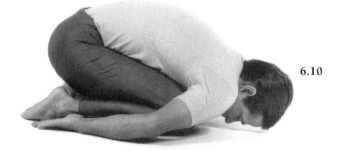

6.10

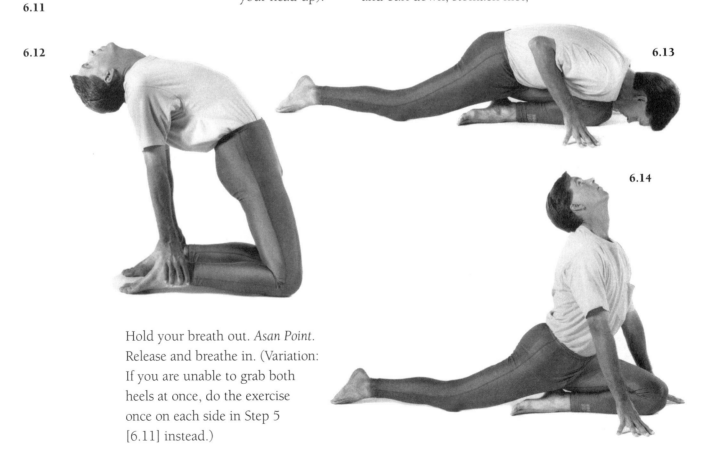

5. Camel Pose. Come up on your knees, separate your knees slightly, arch your back and grab your left heel with your left hand (6.11). Breathe normally. Do this once on each side to warm up. Then reach back and grab both heels (6.12). Let your head gently fall back as you breathe out (unless you have a disk problem in your upper back or neck, in which case keep your head up).

6.11

6. Pigeon Pose. From the Camel Pose, bend forward briefly into the Baby Pose, then sit up and slide your right leg back so you are sitting on your left heel. Your right leg should be as straight as possible, knee to the floor. Place your hands on either side of your left knee and your forehead on the floor (6.13). Breathe out completely, then breathe in as you curl up, head first, then chest, then stomach, curling back as far as you can. You can press up on your fingertips for an extra stretch. Look up toward your forehead (6.14). Hold your breath in. *Asan Point.* Breathe out and curl down, stomach first,

6.12

6.13

6.14

Hold your breath out. *Asan Point.* Release and breathe in. (Variation: If you are unable to grab both heels at once, do the exercise once on each side in Step 5 [6.11] instead.)

keeping your head and eyes up until your head reaches the floor. Repeat three times, then push yourself up on your fists, straighten your arms, relax your back, and stare at one spot on the floor about three feet in front of you (6.15). Breathe out and hold. *Asan Point.* Breathe in as you release the position.

Transition: Push up into the V position (6.8), sliding your left leg back and bringing your right knee forward. Repeat the Pigeon Pose on the right side, then rest in the Baby Pose (6.10).

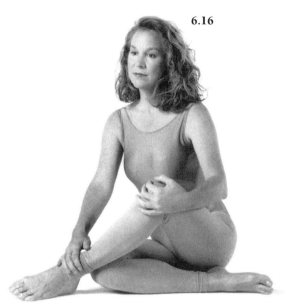

6.16

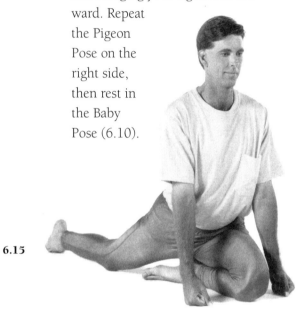

6.15

7. Spine Twist. (a) From the Baby Pose, sit up and slide your hips to the right. Pick up your left foot and carry it across your right knee. Pull your right foot in close to your body (6.16). Turn toward the left and bring your right arm over your left knee. With your right elbow, press your left knee back as far as it will go, then straighten your right arm

and grasp the left big toe (see Chapter 4, photo 4.35). If you can't reach your toe, grasp your left ankle or right knee instead. (b) Bring your left hand close in to your body, fingers pointed in, and straighten the arm. Straighten your back, breathe in looking forward, then breathe out as you twist toward the left as far as you can. Look at a spot on the wall just above eye level (6.17). Hold your breath out. *Asan Point.* Repeat on the opposite side.

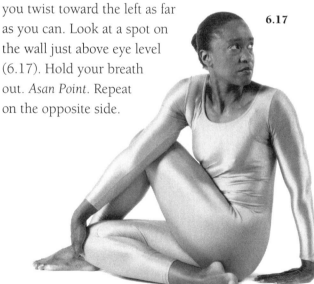

6.17

8. Seated Sun Pose. (a) Bring both legs straight out in front of you and flex your toes. Sit straight, breathe out with arms at sides, then breathe in as you raise your arms in a wide circle to the sides and overhead. Press your palms together, look up, and stretch from the rib cage (6.18). Hold your breath in. *Asan Point.*
(b) Breathe out as you bend forward, tucking your chin toward your chest. If you are limber enough to reach your toes and still bend your elbows, grasp your toes as shown in the close-up (6.20). (If you cannot reach your toes comfortably, grasp your ankles, calves, or knees firmly with both hands.) Pull your torso toward your legs (remember to pull by bending, your arms, not by pushing with your lower back). Hold your breath out (6.19). *Asan Point.*

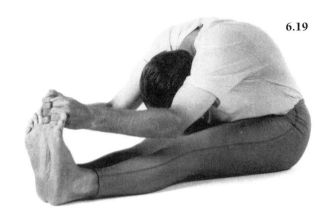

6.19

Release and breathe in, bringing your arms to the sides and over your head again. Stretch and look up as before. Breathe out and bring your arms back down to your sides. Repeat three times.

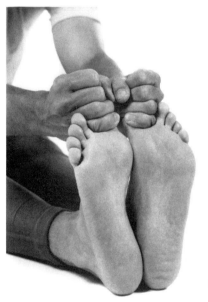

6.20

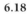

6.18

9. "Telephone" Pose. This is a limbering exercise for knees and hips. (a) Start by gently massaging your knees using the palms of both hands (6.21). The aim is not to apply great pressure but to increase warmth. Massage both knees for several seconds. (b) Now, starting with both legs outstretched, gently pick up your left foot and place it on your right thigh as high as possible.

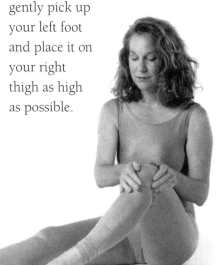

6.21

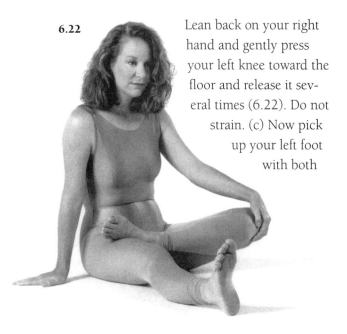

6.22 Lean back on your right hand and gently press your left knee toward the floor and release it several times (6.22). Do not strain. (c) Now pick up your left foot with both hands and gently bring it up toward your right ear (6.23). Do not strain. Lower the foot back on top of your right thigh for the Alternate Seated Sun Pose.

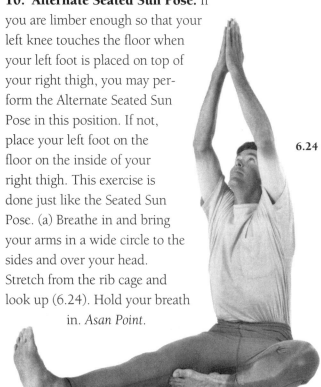

6.23

10. Alternate Seated Sun Pose. If you are limber enough so that your left knee touches the floor when your left foot is placed on top of your right thigh, you may perform the Alternate Seated Sun Pose in this position. If not, place your left foot on the floor on the inside of your right thigh. This exercise is done just like the Seated Sun Pose. (a) Breathe in and bring your arms in a wide circle to the sides and over your head. Stretch from the rib cage and look up (6.24). Hold your breath in. *Asan Point.*

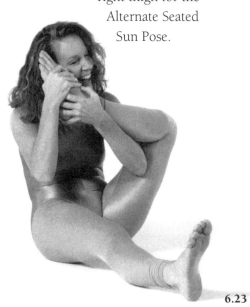

6.24

(b) Breathe out and bend forward over your outstretched leg, keeping your toes flexed. If you are limber enough to reach your toes and still bend your elbows, grasp your toes as shown in the close-up (6.26). (If you cannot reach your toes comfortably, grasp your ankle, calf, or knee firmly with both hands.) Pull your torso gently toward your right leg (6.25).

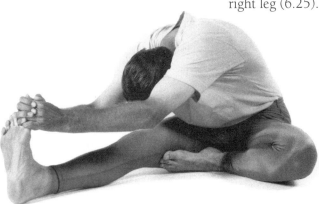

6.25

Hold your breath out. *Asan Point.* Breathe in and raise your arms to the sides and over your head again. Stretch and look up. Hold your breath in. *Asan Point.* Breathe out and lower. Repeat three times.

Transition: Change to opposite side (right foot on left thigh) and repeat Steps 9 and 10 on that side.

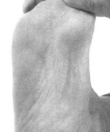

6.26

11. Hero Pose. (a) Start with both legs straight in front of you. Bend your left knee and place your left foot on the inside of your right thigh. Gently bend your right leg back to the right and curl your right foot around your right hip (6.27). (If you are limber enough, you may lift your left foot on top of your right thigh [6.28]; bring your knees closer together in this variation.) Place your right hand on the outside of your right knee, and your left hand on the

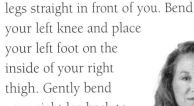

6.27

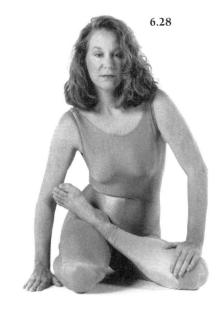

6.28

floor just above your left knee. (b) Breathe in and straighten your spine. Breathe out and bend forward, keeping your hips on the floor and bending your head and upper body toward the floor between your knees (6.29). Breathe in and come up again, then breathe out and bend, bringing your head a little closer to your right knee.

6.29

Breathe in and come up, then breathe out and bend a third time, bringing your head as close to your right knee as possible. (As your limberness increases, you will be able to lay your chest on your right thigh.) Close your eyes and hold your breath out. *Asan Point.* Breathe in and come up. Switch to the opposite side by first lifting your left foot off your thigh. Pick up your right foot and *gently* swing it around to the front, letting your right knee rest on the floor. Then lift your left foot and swing it around back to curl around your left hip. Bring your right foot to the inside of your left thigh, or lift it on top of your left thigh, and repeat the exercise. This time you will be bending your head close to your left knee instead of your right.

12. Tortoise Stretch. (a) Straighten your legs and separate them as far as possible. Straighten your back and breathe in as you raise your arms in a wide circle to the sides and over your head (6.30). (b) Breathe out as you bend forward, reaching for your toes with each hand (6.31). If you can reach your toes easily, grasp the big toe as in the Alternate Seated Sun Pose (see 6.26); if not, grasp ankles or calves. Hold your breath out. *Asan Point.* Breathe in and raise your arms back over your head, then breathe out and lower your arms to your sides. Repeat three times.

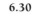

6.30

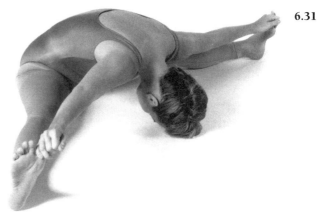

6.31

13. Lotus Pose. This exercise and the three that follow should not be attempted if you have back problems. Instead, skip to the Alternate Toe Touch (Step 17). After performing all the limbering exercises above, try the Lotus by gently lifting both feet, one at a time, and placing them on top of the opposite thigh (6.32). Never force yourself into this position or hold it in pain. If you are comfortable in the Lotus position, try sitting in this pose while you do your breathing exercises. When the pose becomes comfortable, you may attempt the next three exercises.

14. Lotus Fish Pose. With your legs in the Lotus position, gently lower your elbows to the floor (6.33), arch your back, and slowly lower your head to the floor. Place your hands

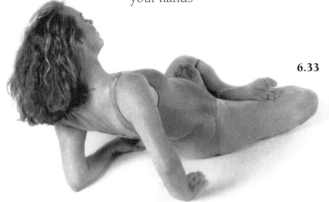

6.33

6.32

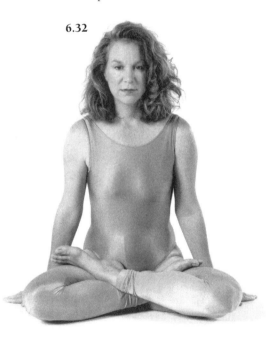

palms down next to your body (6.34) or, if you are quite comfortable and limber in this position, grasp the big toes of each foot with your fingers. Look up through your forehead and breathe out. Hold the breath out. *Asan Point.* Breathe in and release, lie flat, and rest. (Note: If you are unable to hold the Lotus Pose throughout all three exercises, release, massage your knees, shake your legs out, and rest after each one.)

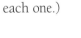

6.34

15. Lotus Shoulder Stand. (a) From a seated position in the Lotus, roll back onto your shoulders, bringing your knees to your forehead and supporting your back with both hands (6.35). (b) Slowly straighten your legs and then straighten your back by pushing forward with your hands so your weight moves to the back of your neck

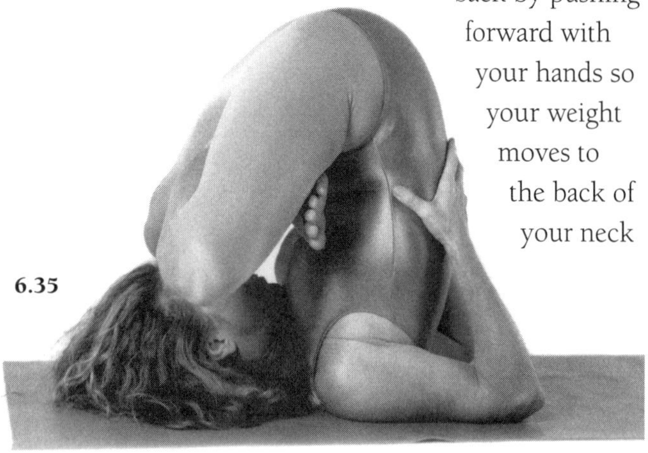

6.35

(6.36). Stare at one spot on the ceiling and do not turn your head. Breathe out and hold your breath out. *Asan Point*. Breathe in and roll back down into a seated position. Bend your head forward and rest a moment.

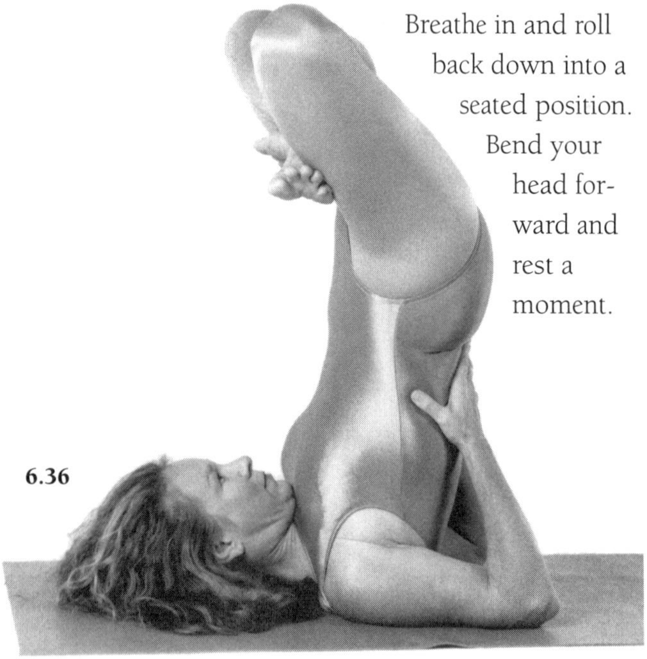

6.36

16. Lotus Cobra Pose. Do not attempt this exercise unless you are comfortable in the Lotus Fish Pose. Transition: (a) From a seated position in the Lotus, push yourself up on your knees and support yourself on your hands (6.37) as you lower yourself onto your stomach. (b) Place your hands close

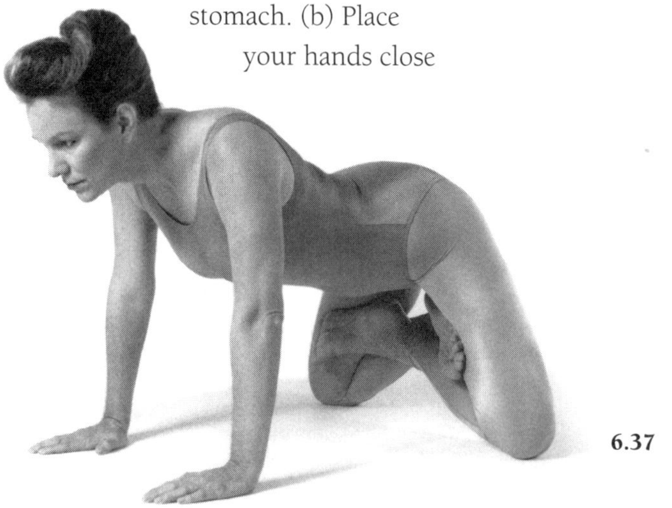

6.37

in to your body, palms down, elbows raised. Place your forehead on the floor (6.38). (c) Breathe out completely, then breathe in as you curl your head and torso up and back, looking up through your forehead (6.39). Hold your breath in. *Asan Point*. Breathe out as you curl down, stomach first, then chest, and then

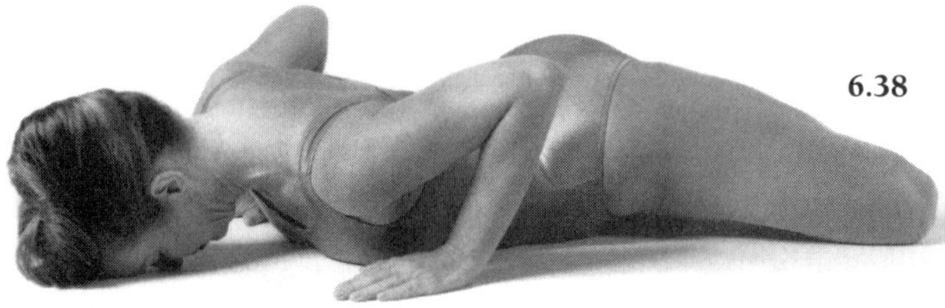

6.38

6.39

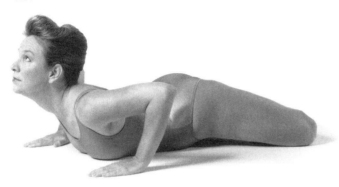

head and eyes. Repeat three times. You may need to rest between each repetition.

Transition: Push yourself up on your knees and gently lower yourself to a seated position. Release the Lotus Pose, massage both knees, and slowly straighten them. Shake both legs, then rest in the Corpse Pose (6.40).

17. Alternate Toe Touch. Lie on your back with arms overhead and legs together. Breathe out. Breathe in as you lift your left arm and left leg and reach for your big toe (you can also lift the opposite arm and leg for a different stretch). If you can, grasp the toe with your thumb and fore-finger (6.41). (If you are very limber, you can reach around your big toe with your hand, as in the Alternate Seated Sun Pose [6.26].) Another way to stretch into this position is to first bend the left knee, grasp the toe, and carefully straighten the leg as far as you can without strain. Repeat once on each side.

6.40

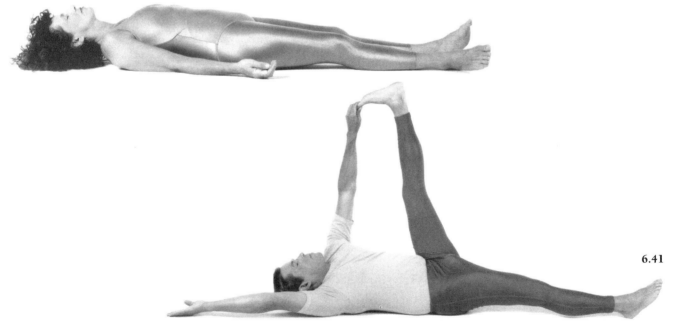

6.41

18. Wheel. Prepare for this exercise by practicing the **Easy Bridge**: Bend your knees and separate your legs and feet several inches; place your arms at your sides, palms down or grasping your ankles, as shown. Breathe in, then breathe out as you lift your hips, arching your back and tucking your chin into your chest (6.42). Hold your breath out. *Asan Point.* Repeat three times.

sides, and rest in the Corpse Pose (6.40).

End the Flexibility Routine with Complete Breath, Alternate Nostril Breath, and fifteen to thirty minutes of meditation, either seated or lying down (see Chapter 2).

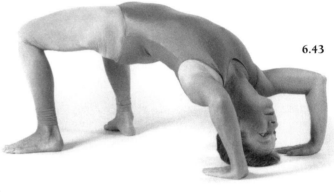

6.43

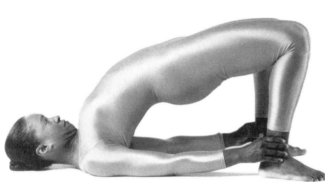

6.42

For the Wheel, place your hands next to your head, fingers pointing toward your feet. Breathe in and push up so you are resting on your head (6.43). If you can, continue pushing up into the full position (6.44). Hold your breath in. *Asan Point.* Breathe out and lower your body to the floor, straighten your legs, bring your arms down to your

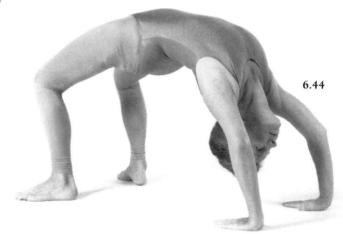

6.44

7

Focus

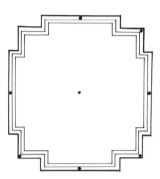

*One representation of the emotional makeup of a
human being*

Most of the time our minds are split among many different things. The multiple demands of work, family, and society seem to pull at us from all directions. Often we feel as if we are spending all our time reacting to these external demands instead of listening to the creative voice of our inner self. In many cases, the problem is not so much the number of external demands as it is our inability to focus easily.

It is very difficult to put your attention on something and hold that point as long as you wish. If you are lucky or persevering enough to experience this rare quality, creative thought then becomes a sweet, free-flowing experience. Oftentimes we find ourselves seeking creativity under extreme stress, when it can hardly flourish. The effort becomes a hard, cruel, futile whipping of oneself. The prime climate for the bright glow of creativity is silence.

Silence is the supreme goal of concentration. It is a rare experience in the world of work and society, but it can be developed. Every time you practice the Asan Point (see "The Asan Point" in Chapter 1) with your Yoga exercises you give a momentary gift of silence to your mind. Your regular daily meditation practice brings a longer period of healing silence to your mind. If you do these two things you will very quickly enjoy great progress in directing thought toward one thing—or toward no thought. Breathing techniques are another way to begin to pare down the number of thoughts in your mind at one time. As you practice the breath exercises, you will notice the automatic quieting of other thoughts. It is practically impossible to entertain a number of scattered thoughts in your mind while focusing on the breath.

Use these three techniques—Asan Point in exercises, breathing techniques, and meditation—together whenever you can for the strongest, quickest results. If you have to practice asans at one time and breathing and meditation at another time, I suggest keeping the breathing and meditation together. You can always give yourself some additional practice by doing your breathing exercises at odd times, such as waiting in a doctor's office, during traffic tie-ups, waiting for people who are late, and so on. A side benefit is that time passes very quickly and boredom has no chance to set in.

In this chapter you will learn two routines that sharpen your focusing skills. The Concentration Routine includes fewer exercises than other routines, but they are held longer. The Balance Routine consists entirely of exercises that require physical balance in addition to mental concentration.

The Concentration Routine

In this routine, try to hold the Asan Point for several seconds. If you are vegetarian, you may do some of the asans, as indicated, with one or two physical "locks," or muscle contractions, which are meant to intensify the energies of the body. The first lock involves pressing the chin into the triangular space at the joint of the collarbones with the breath held out (*jalandara bandha*). The second lock involves breathing in deeply, then breathing out and contracting the rectal muscles with the breath held out (*mula bandha*). If you are not vegetarian, you should not use these locks with these exercises. Instead, do the routine as described without the locks.

At the places marked *Asan Point*, try to hold the position for a few seconds with body in pose, breath held (in or out, depending on the exercise), eyes focused, and mind silent. (For more on the Asan Point, see Chapter 1.) Hold the Asan Point only as long as it is comfortable.

1. Standing Sun Pose. (a) Stand with feet together, arms at your sides. Your knees should be straight but not locked. Breathe out. Breathe in as you raise your arms in a wide circle out to the sides and overhead. Stretch and look up at your hands (7.1). Hold your breath in. *Asan Point.* (b) Breathe out as you bend forward from the waist, keeping your hands together and your head between your arms (7.2). (c) Hold your breath out as you grasp your ankles or calves firmly, bend your elbows, tuck your chin, and pull

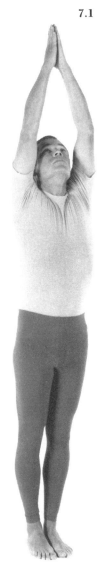

7.1

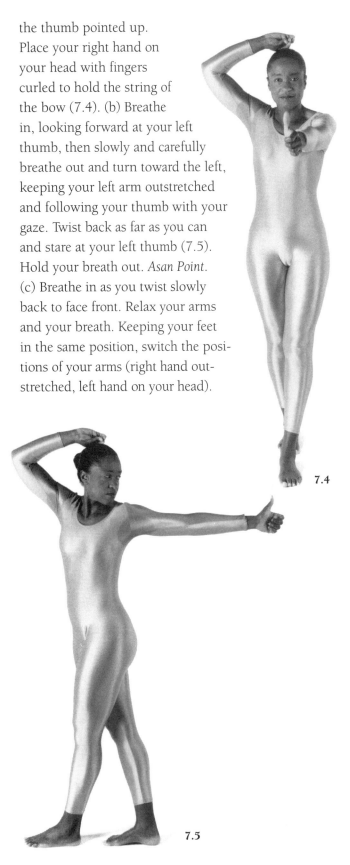

your torso toward your legs (7.3) (be sure to pull by bending your elbows instead of straining your lower back). Keep your knees straight but not locked. Tuck your chin into your throat and contract your rectal muscles. Hold your breath out. *Asan Point.* (Note: If you have back or neck problems, bend only halfway down, and do not pull your torso in.) Release and breathe in as you slowly straighten, bringing your arms in a wide circle out to the sides and over your head. Look up and stretch as in Step 1(a). Hold your breath in. *Asan Point.* Breathe out and slowly lower your arms to your sides. Repeat three times.

2. Archer Pose.
(a) Place your left foot directly in front of the right, both pointed straight ahead. If you feel unsteady in this position, you may separate your feet slightly at first, but both should point forward. Extend your left arm straight ahead and position the hand as if you were holding a bow, with the thumb pointed up. Place your right hand on your head with fingers curled to hold the string of the bow (7.4). (b) Breathe in, looking forward at your left thumb, then slowly and carefully breathe out and turn toward the left, keeping your left arm outstretched and following your thumb with your gaze. Twist back as far as you can and stare at your left thumb (7.5). Hold your breath out. *Asan Point.* (c) Breathe in as you twist slowly back to face front. Relax your arms and your breath. Keeping your feet in the same position, switch the positions of your arms (right hand outstretched, left hand on your head).

7.2

7.3

7.4

7.5

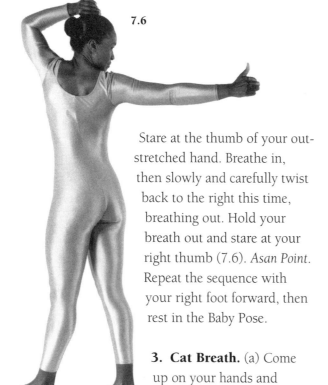

7.6

Stare at the thumb of your out-stretched hand. Breathe in, then slowly and carefully twist back to the right this time, breathing out. Hold your breath out and stare at your right thumb (7.6). *Asan Point.* Repeat the sequence with your right foot forward, then rest in the Baby Pose.

3. Cat Breath. (a) Come up on your hands and knees. Breathe in as you arch your back and look up toward the ceiling (7.7). Hold your breath in. *Asan Point.* (b) Breathe out as you round your back, tuck your chin into your chest, pull in and up

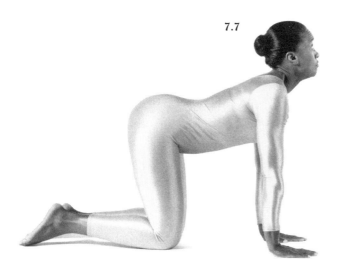

7.7

on your stomach, and contract your rectal muscles (7.8). Hold your breath out. *Asan Point.*

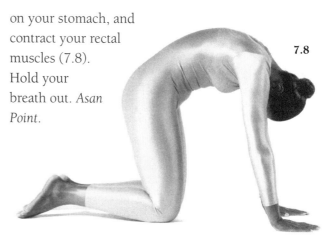

7.8

4. Peacock Pose. This is a very strenuous exercise that should not be done by women during the menstrual cycle or at any time during pregnancy. (a) Start by sitting on your feet. Separate your knees and place your hands on the floor between your legs as far back as you can, palms down and fingers facing backward. Bring your elbows together (7.9). (b) Lean forward, round your back, and position your arms so that your abdomen and chest are resting on the backs of your upper arms. Slide one leg back straight (7.10), rest your head on the

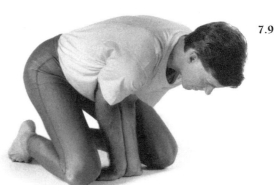

7.9

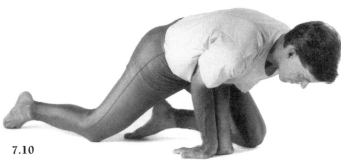

7.10

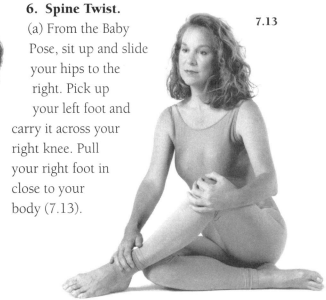

7.13

floor, then slide the other leg back. (c) For the completed pose, breathe in, lift your head and look forward, then gently touch off with your toes until your legs are straight (7.11).

6. Spine Twist.

(a) From the Baby Pose, sit up and slide your hips to the right. Pick up your left foot and carry it across your right knee. Pull your right foot in close to your body (7.13).

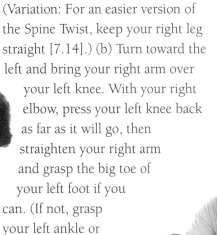

7.14

7.11

(Variation: For an easier version of the Spine Twist, keep your right leg straight [7.14].) (b) Turn toward the left and bring your right arm over your left knee. With your right elbow, press your left knee back as far as it will go, then straighten your right arm and grasp the big toe of your left foot if you can. (If not, grasp your left ankle or your right calf

Hold your breath in. *Asan Point.* Breathe out and release.

5. Rest in the **Baby Pose** (7.12).

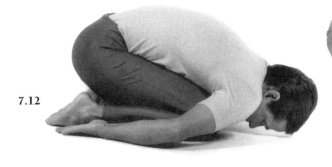

7.12

or knee instead.) (c) Bring your left hand in close to the base of your spine, fingers pointed in, and straighten your arm. Straighten your back, breathe in looking forward, then breathe out as you twist toward the left as far as you can. Breathe naturally. Look at a spot on the wall just above eye level (7.15). Hold your breath out. *Asan Point.* Breathe in and release, then repeat on the opposite side.

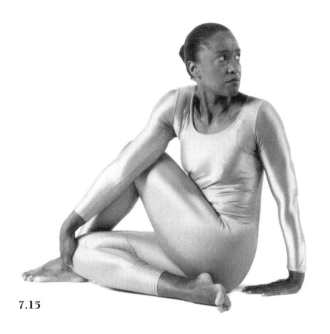

7.15

7. Hero Pose. (a) Bring both legs straight out in front of you. Carefully bend your right leg back and curl your right foot around your right hip. Bend your left knee and place your right foot on the inside of the left thigh (7.16). (Variation: If you are limber enough, you may lift your left foot on top of your right thigh

[7.17]; bring your knees closer together in this variation.) Place your right hand on the outside of your right knee, and your left hand on the floor just above your left knee. (b) Breathe in and straighten your back. Breathe out and bend forward, bending your head and upper body toward the floor between your knees (7.18). Your hips remain on the floor. Hold your breath out, tuck your chin into your chest, and contract your rectal muscles. *Asan Point.* Breathe in and come up again, then breathe out and bend, bringing your head a little closer to your right knee. Hold your breath out, tuck your chin into your chest, and contract your rectal muscles. *Asan Point.* Breathe in and come up, then breathe out and bend a third time, bringing your head as close to your right knee as possible.

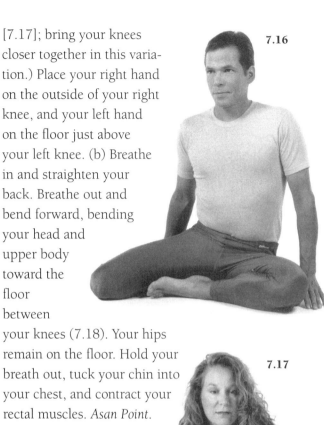

7.16

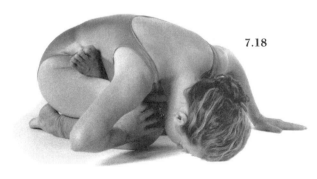

7.17

7.18

(As your limberness increases, you will be able to lay your chest on your right thigh.) Close your eyes and hold your breath out. *Asan Point*.

Transition: Switch to the opposite side by first lifting your left foot off your thigh to position 7(a). Pick up your right foot and *gently* swing it around to the front, letting your right knee rest on the floor. Then lift your left foot and swing it around back to curl around your left hip. Bring your right foot to the inside of your left thigh (or lift it on top of your left thigh) and repeat the exercise. This time you will be bending your head close to your left knee instead of your right.

8. Diamond Pose. (a) Sit with the soles of your feet together, knees relaxed outward, hands clasped around your toes (7.19). (b) Breathe in and straighten your back, then breathe out and bend forward, bringing your

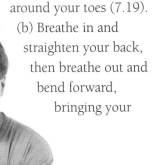

7.19

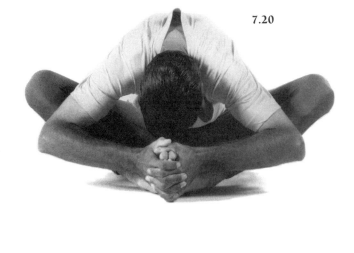

7.20

head toward your feet and letting your elbows fall outside your knees. Hold your breath out, tuck your chin into your throat, and contract your rectal muscles (7.20). Hold your breath out. *Asan Point*. Breathe in and release.

9. Locust Pose. Lie on your stomach with your chin to the floor and your arms at your sides. Make your hands into fists and press the *top* of the fist (thumb and forefinger edge) into the floor. Breathe in and hold your breath as you lift one leg as high as possible in back, pressing down with your fists into the floor (7.21). Keep the knee of the lifted leg straight—you are lifting from the hip. Breathe out and lower the leg. Repeat three times with each leg. The full Locust Pose requires a bit more strength. From the starting position,

7.21

7.22

10. Cobra Pose. (a) Bring your hands close in to your body under your armpits, with elbows raised, and your forehead to the floor (7.23). Breathe out. (b) Breathe in as you first curl your head back, then lift your chest off the floor, then your stomach, using your back muscles more than your arms. Keep your eyes focused between your eyebrows (7.24). Hold your breath in. *Asan Point*. Breathe out as you curl down in reverse: stomach first, then chest, then head, bringing your forehead back to the floor. Repeat three times.

breathe out completely, then breathe in and raise both legs, keeping your knees straight and lifting from the hip, as high as you can (7.22). Hold your breath in. *Asan Point*. Breathe out and bring legs back down, then rest on your stomach.

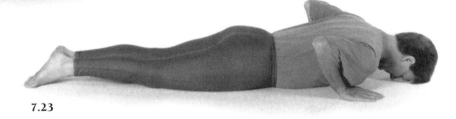

7.23

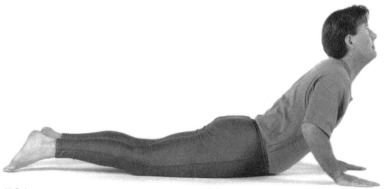

7.24

11. Shoulder Stand. (a) Start in a seated position with knees drawn up and arms around your knees. Roll back onto your shoulders, bringing your knees to your forehead, and support your lower back with your hands (7.25). (b) Slowly straighten your legs toward the ceiling, pushing forward with your hands as far as you can comfortably to shift your weight onto the back of your neck (7.26).

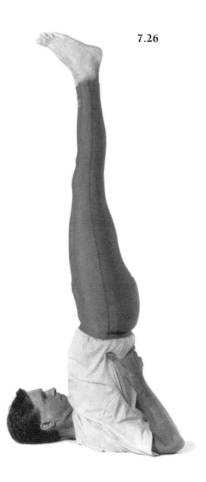

7.26

7.25

Look up at your feet. Breathe out and hold your breath out. *Asan Point.* Breathe in and bend your knees, bringing them back to your forehead (7.25), then roll forward into a cross-legged position (7.27), and then rest a few moments with head and arms forward. Do not do this exercise if you have disk problems in your neck. For those with chronic back problems, the Easy Bridge (see Chapter 6, page 92) is an easier inverted exercise. You can also benefit from simply lying on your back on the floor with your legs resting on a chair seat or bed.

Finish the Concentration Routine with the Complete Breath, the Soft Bellows Breath, and the Rising

Breath. Meditate seated or lying down for fifteen to thirty minutes. For a review of meditation, see Chapter 2.

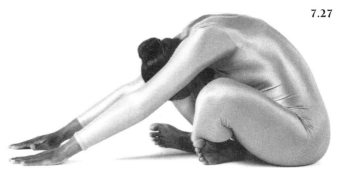

7.27

THE MEANING OF *ASAN*

There are eighty-four hundreds of thousands of asanas described by Shiva. The postures are as many in number as there are numbers of species of living creatures in this universe. Among them eighty-four are the best, and among these eighty-four, thirty-two have been found useful for mankind in this world.

(*Gheranda Samhita*)

The word *asan* can be interpreted in many ways. Here are a few examples from a Sanskrit–English dictionary published over a hundred years ago:

1. Sitting in peculiar posture according to the custom of devotees.
2. The manner of sitting forming part of the eightfold observances of ascetics.
3. The part where the driver sits.
4. Maintaining a post against an enemy.
5. The withers of an elephant.
6. To make a seat out of anything—even a lotus.

These are only a few of the meanings of the word. As you can see, this is a far deeper interpretation than most Americans have been given in the practice of Yoga exercise. I find it delightful to consider all of these possibilities while doing asans.

The Balance Routine

Focusing exercises are not usually thought of as requiring great strength, but the truth is that they put great strain on the nervous system. For this reason, most people avoid intense concentration because it becomes uncomfortable. To become completely comfortable in effortless, one-pointed concentration, you will need to practice daily using both your mind and your body. The Balance Routine is the best way to build this skill. Although all exercises done with the Asan Point will increase your ability for strong, directed thought, the Balance Routine will give you the quickest results.

Balance poses are the best indicators of the health and strength of your nervous system. Your nervous system reflects how you are handling the stress in your life, the adequacy of your diet, and your emotional stability. You can tell the status of your nervous system by how soon your body starts to shake after you have taken a balance position. Some days you will notice more steadiness than others, of course, but if you notice this shaking several days in a row, you should seriously examine your lifestyle and see if you can make some changes to build up your strength and stamina. Special care should be given to including adequate B complex vitamins in your diet.

Because this is such a demanding routine, rest for a few moments after each exercise, in one of the rest positions described in Chapter 2. Practice standing exercises with a sturdy chair nearby for support.

At the places marked *Asan Point*, try to hold the position for a few seconds with body in pose, breath held (in or out, depending on the exercise), eyes focused, and mind silent. (For more on the Asan Point, see "The Asan Point" in Chapter 1.) Hold the Asan Point only as long as it is comfortable.

1. Tree Pose. From a standing position, lift your right foot and place it on the inside of your left thigh (7.28). Relax the leg to help hold your foot in position. Bare feet will

also help. Steady yourself by gazing at one spot on the wall or floor (without bending your neck), and breathe in as you raise your arms slowly over your head, straighten your arms, and place your palms together (7.29). Hold your breath in. *Asan Point.*

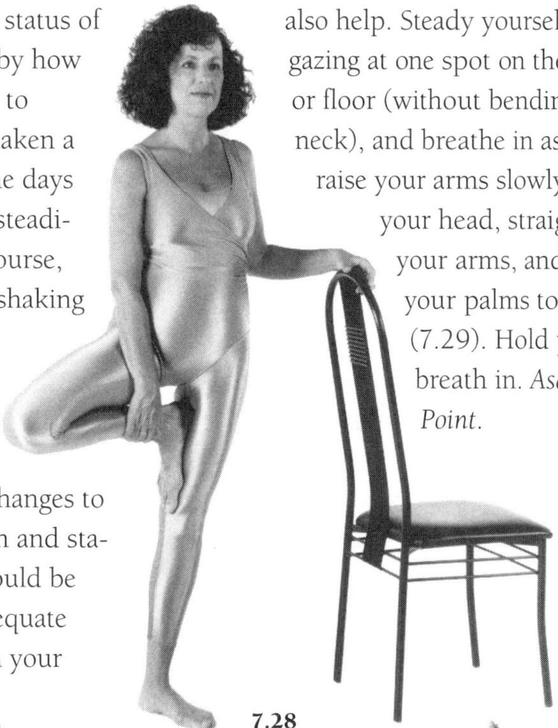

7.28

Breathe out and bring arms and leg down slowly. If you are limber enough, you may place your foot on top of your thigh (7.30).

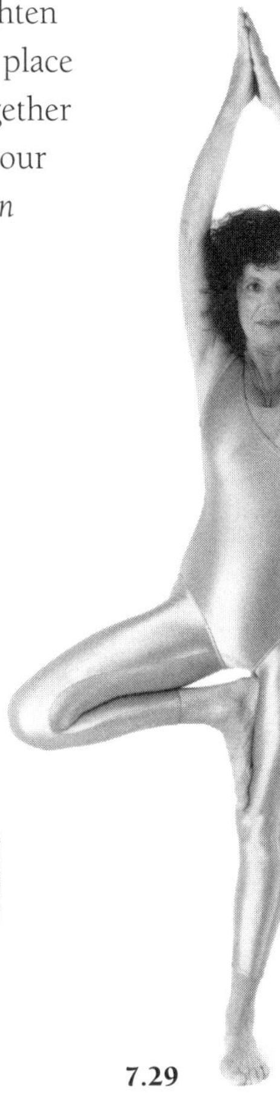

7.29

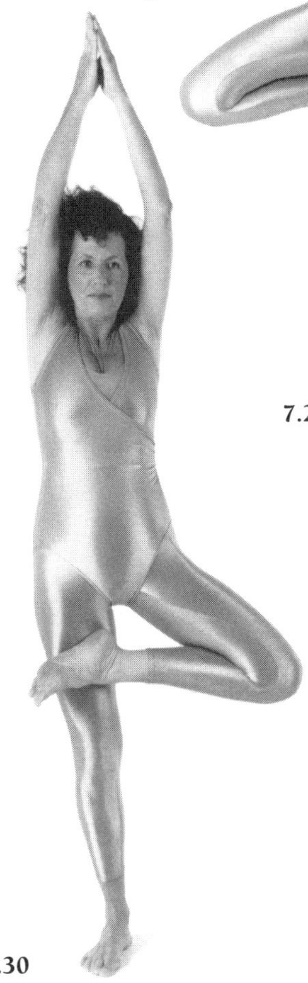

7.30

2. Eagle Pose. Stare at one spot on the floor for balance (or stare at the bindu point in the diagram at the beginning of the chapter). Bend your left leg slightly. Wrap your right leg over and behind the left leg (if you can't reach behind the leg, just go as far as you can). When you're steady, bend your torso and place your *left* elbow on your *right* knee. Then place your right elbow *inside* your left elbow, turn your hands toward each other, and clasp your fingers. Breathe out as you bend your head so your forehead rests on your hands (7.31). Hold your breath out. *Asan Point.* Slowly breathe in, untwist, and switch sides.

7.31

3. Dancer Pose and Extension. (a) From a standing position, bend one leg and grasp your foot with the opposite hand (7.32). Throughout the exercise, steady yourself by fixing your gaze on one spot on the wall in front of you. (b) Slowly move into the completed Dancer Pose by raising your free arm straight up toward the ceiling next to your ear and pulling your lifted leg *up* and *back* as far as possible without strain. Keep your supporting leg straight and keep your gaze focused on one spot (7.33). Breathe in and hold your breath in. *Asan Point.* (c) Maintaining

7.32

your gaze, slowly breathe out and lower your body into the extended position (7.34). Keep your lifted leg as far up and back as possible. Your free arm extends straight ahead. Your supporting leg remains straight. Stare at one spot for balance. Don't strain. Hold for a moment, then breathe in, come back to a standing position, and switch sides.

7.33

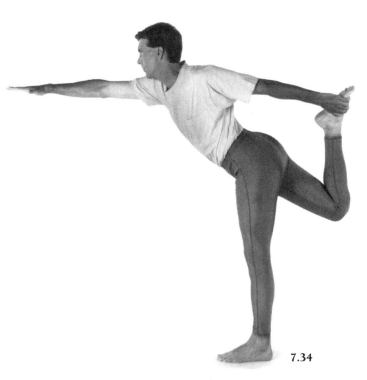

7.34

4. T Pose. When you are first learning this position, stand about three to four feet from a chair or other support. Lean forward and hold on to the support with both hands. Lift your left leg in back as high as you can (ideally, parallel to the floor). Keep your right (supporting) leg straight. Your torso and left leg should be in a straight line parallel to the floor. Keep your neck straight, breathe naturally, and look at a spot on the floor (7.35). When you feel steady, release your grip on the support and place your palms together. Relax your breath (7.36). If you are very steady, you can try looking forward at your hands. Repeat Step 4 on the opposite side.

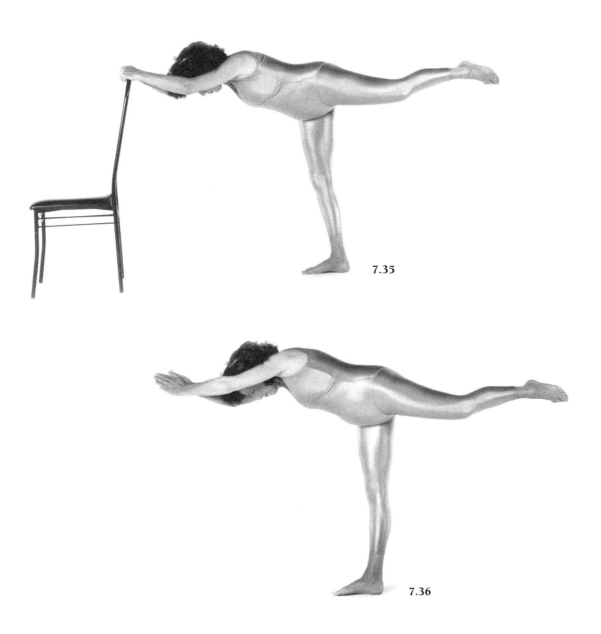

7.35

7.36

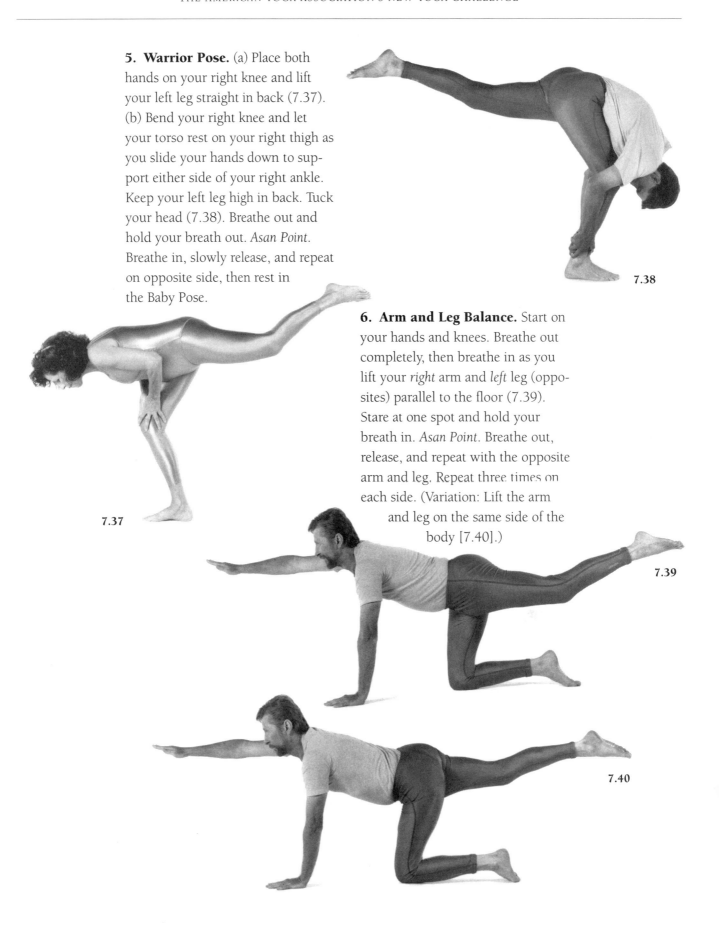

5. Warrior Pose. (a) Place both hands on your right knee and lift your left leg straight in back (7.37). (b) Bend your right knee and let your torso rest on your right thigh as you slide your hands down to support either side of your right ankle. Keep your left leg high in back. Tuck your head (7.38). Breathe out and hold your breath out. *Asan Point.* Breathe in, slowly release, and repeat on opposite side, then rest in the Baby Pose.

7.38

7.37

6. Arm and Leg Balance. Start on your hands and knees. Breathe out completely, then breathe in as you lift your *right* arm and *left* leg (opposites) parallel to the floor (7.39). Stare at one spot and hold your breath in. *Asan Point.* Breathe out, release, and repeat with the opposite arm and leg. Repeat three times on each side. (Variation: Lift the arm and leg on the same side of the body [7.40].)

7.39

7.40

7. Bow Variation. Start on hands and knees. Reach back with your left hand and grasp your right foot. Stare at one spot on the floor for balance as you breathe in and lift your foot up and away from your body as far as possible (7.41). Hold your breath in. *Asan Point.* Breathe out, release slowly, and switch sides. Repeat three times on each side.

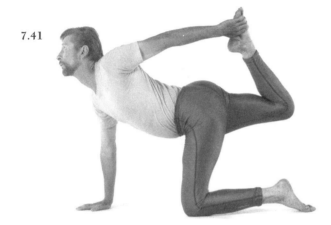

7.41

8. Crow Pose. Squat on your toes, separate your knees, and place your hands on the floor between your knees about a foot apart. Bend your elbows and place the inside joint of your knees on your elbows (you'll have to lift your hips slightly to do this). Carefully lean forward, resting your bent knees on the back of your elbows, until your feet come off the floor (7.42). Breathe out and stare at one spot on the floor. Hold your breath out. *Asan Point.*

7.42

9. Side Crow Pose. Squat on your toes, knees together. Move your right foot forward several inches. Turn toward the right and place both hands on the floor, fingers facing right, as close in to your body as possible (7.43). Lift your hips, bend your elbows, and shift your body weight onto the backs of your upper arms; your right hip will rest on your right arm and your right thigh on your left arm (7.44). Carefully lean forward until you are balanced and your feet come off the floor. Straighten your legs as much as you can (7.45). Stare at one spot on the floor. Breathe out and hold your breath out. *Asan Point.* Breathe in, release slowly, and repeat on the other side.

7.43

7.44

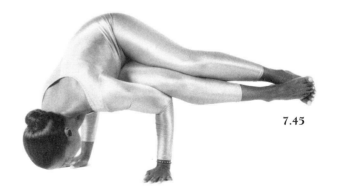

7.45

10. Rest in the **Baby Pose** (7.46).

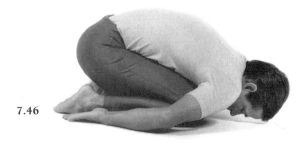

7.46

11. Two preparatory exercises will help you limber up for the One-Legged Sage Pose:

Ankle Stretch. Sit on your feet and lift your knees, leaning back on your hands to stretch the tops of your feet (7.47). Lower and repeat several times. Breathe naturally.

Hip and Knee Stretch. Be sure you are exercising on a soft blanket or foam mat. Sit on your right foot and lift your left foot on top of your right thigh as if you were beginning the Hero Pose (see Chapter 6). Bring your knees closer together. Push yourself carefully up on your knees, maintaining the position, and try to straighten your torso. Your right calf remains on the floor for balance. When you feel steady, breathe in as you straighten your arms over your

7.47

head and place your palms together (7.48). Stare at one spot on the wall or floor in front of you. Hold your breath in. *Asan Point*. Breathe out, release slowly, and repeat on the opposite side.

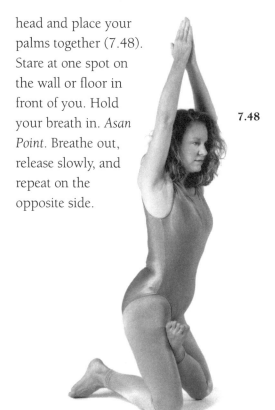

7.48

12. One-Legged Sage Pose. Do not attempt this exercise unless you can easily do the preparatory exercises in Step 11 and the Hero Pose with your foot on your thigh, and you have no joint problems in either knee. (a) Sit on your right foot and place your left ankle high on your right thigh. Lean forward on your hands and knees, and lift your left knee off the floor. Reach under your left (lifted) ankle with your right elbow so it rests on the back of your right upper arm (7.49).

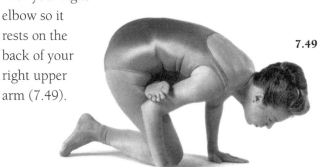

7.49

Your hand rests on the floor next to your right knee. (b) Reach under your left knee with your left elbow so the knee rests on the back of your left upper arm (7.50). (c) Breathe in, slide your right leg back and straighten it as you balance with your weight on your hands and head (7.51). (d) Slowly lift your right leg and head off the floor for the completed pose (7.52). Stare at one spot on the floor in front of you. Hold your breath in. *Asan Point*. Breathe out, release slowly, repeat on the opposite side, and then rest in the Baby Pose.

7.50

13. Shoulder Stand. Do not do this exercise if you have back or neck problems; substitute the Easy Bridge (see page 92). Sit up and roll back onto your shoulders, immediately supporting your back with your hands and keeping your knees bent and touching your forehead (7.53). Slowly straighten your legs toward the ceiling and push your back straighter by using your hands. Stare at the spot between your big toes and breathe out (7.54). Hold your breath out. *Asan Point*. Breathe in and relax your breath.

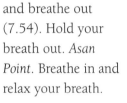

7.53

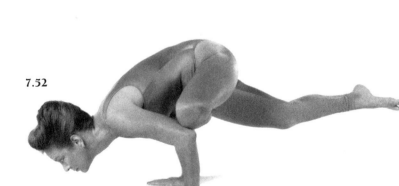

7.51

7.52

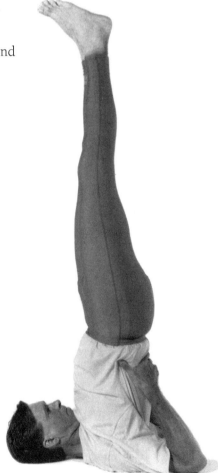

7.54

14. Candle Pose. From the Shoulder Stand, let your back relax slightly so your weight is on your upper back instead of your neck. Carefully lift your arms up along your sides so you are balancing on your back. Stare at one spot on the ceiling and breathe out (7.55). Hold your breath out. *Asan Point*. Breathe in and release.

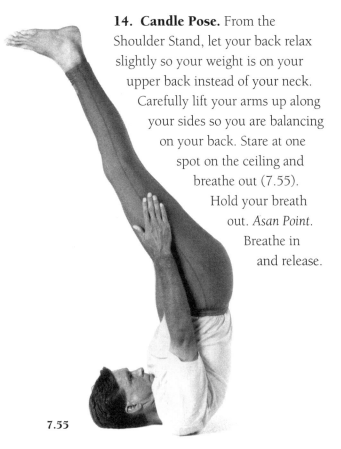

7.55

15. Support your back with your hands, bring your knees back to your forehead, and roll all the way forward to a cross-legged position with your head to the floor (7.56). **Rest** in this position for several moments, then lie on your back and continue resting in the Corpse Pose.

7.56

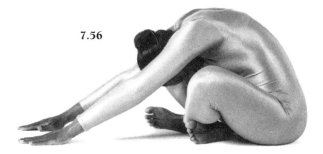

16. Big Sit-up Variation. Sit up and bend your knees. Grasp your toes with both hands, balance on your buttocks (7.57), breathe in, and slowly straighten your legs, keeping a grip on your toes (7.58). Hold your breath in. *Asan Point*. Breathe out and release slowly, then rest in the Corpse Pose.

7.57

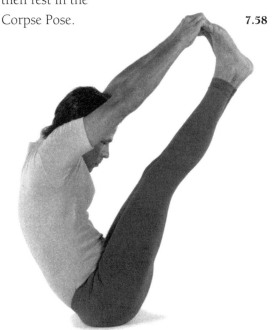

7.58

Finish the Balance Routine with the Complete Breath, Alternate Nostril Breath, and meditation seated or lying down (see Chapter 2).

8
Steadiness

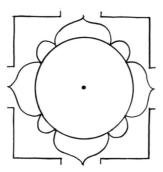

An aspect of Vishnu, the preserver

Advancing Yoga students must perceive themselves as possessing heroic qualities in order to achieve the balance of a powerful individual. A strong, healthy body does not, by itself, necessarily imply sensitivity, depth, spontaneity, and awareness—all essential qualities of a hero. Many times I meet people who look good, only to find as I get to know them that looking good is all they have—very much like an impressive-looking car with a brand-new paint job but a faulty engine. One description of a hero is a person who can take one more step, one more than anyone else. This takes courage, perseverance, emotional strength, and silence. Strength and limberness alone cannot build heroic qualities in a qualified student.

The Emotional Stability Routine, with attention to the Asan Point in each exercise, can help add these vital qualities to your personality while it strengthens your body and protects it from stress. The Asan Point especially is needed to practice silence, which is absolutely necessary in order for new thought patterns to emerge in the mind. Emotional stability training helps you achieve the balance that is needed to face the transforming changes that will occur as you advance in Yoga.

This training will also help you call on reserve forces from within when unexpected stress demands extra strength and stamina. The ability to respond to the extra demand without causing the body pain or depleting its resources is gained only by slow, steady practice.

Ethical behavior is of paramount importance in building this protection from stress. Review the ten ethical guidelines of Yoga (see Chapter 6) and check your adherence to them at the first sign of stress. I used to keep the list on my refrigerator door so it was always in sight, and I learned to connect my emotional stability to these concepts. I have since observed in my students that when they are upset, it is usually because they have moved away from these ethical principles in some way.

The Emotional Stability Routine

This routine is one of the most effective ways to build resistance to stress. Our physical and emotional reactions to stress tend to lodge in the body in the form of tight muscles and constricted breathing patterns, particularly in the stomach, chest, face, and upper back. As we go through our day, we can't always say or do what we want, so stress often goes unacknowledged. Many everyday situations cause us to feel fear, anxiety, or dread, but we do not allow ourselves to express these feelings, and they don't go away. Instead, they brood and fester in our minds and bodies, creating subtle havoc, which manifests as irritability, moodiness, nagging aches or pains, digestive upset, lost sleep, "ugly fits," and so on. The cumulative effect of this poor handling of stress is a dampening of the immune system, leading to greater vulnerability to disease.

Our first tendency is to blame the source of the stress for how we feel (the boss, the weather, the car, the spouse), but the problem is, rather, our reaction to it. If we can notice our reaction when it happens, we can remain more balanced in stressful situations and build resistance to illness.

The Emotional Stability Routine helps by releasing emotional tension and strengthening the body's natural resilience. Practice it four or five times a week for a strong support to your everyday life. Since it is a strenuous sequence, you may need to start with fewer repetitions and work up to the maximum.

At the places marked *Asan Point*, try to hold the position for a few seconds with body in pose, breath held (in or out, depending on the exercise), eyes focused, and mind silent. (For more on the Asan Point, see "The Asan Point" in Chapter 1.) Hold the Asan Point only as long as it is comfortable.

1. Windmill. Stand with feet separated about three feet (or a comfortable distance) and hands supporting the lower back. Your toes should point forward at all times. Breathe in and swivel to the right, then breathe out as you bend your head toward your right knee (8.1) and across to your left knee. Start to breathe in as you lift up to a standing position (facing left) and swivel to the right to begin your second repetition. Repeat three to six times to the right, then three to six times to the left.

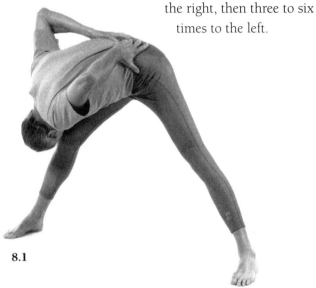

8.1

2. Cobra V-Raise. Bring feet together, bend forward, and walk hands out until you are in the V position (8.2). Tuck your head, push

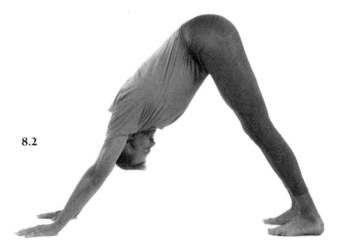

8.2

your heels down to the floor, and breathe out. Hold your breath out. *Asan Point.* Keeping your hands and feet still and arms straight, breathe in as you lower your body and arch your back until you are in the Cobra position. Your head is curled up and back and your eyes are looking straight up to your forehead (8.3). Try to keep your knees from touching the floor. Hold your breath in. *Asan Point.* Breathe out and release. Repeat three to six times.

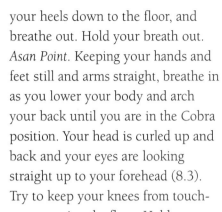

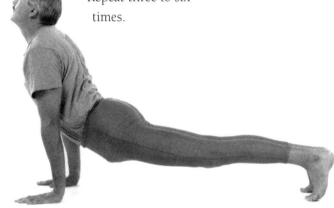

8.3

3. Plank Poses. (a) From the final Cobra position, raise your hips and lower your shoulders until your body is in a straight line supported on your hands and feet. Shift your weight to your right arm and breathe in as you lift your left arm straight in front of you (8.4). Focus your gaze on your outstretched hand. Hold your breath in. *Asan Point.* Breathe out and release. (b) Still supporting yourself on your right arm, breathe

8.4

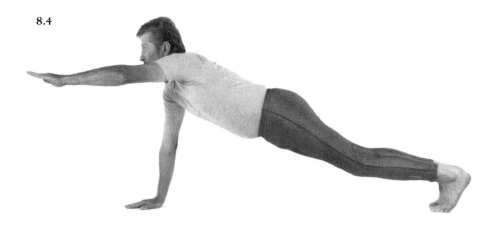

in as you bring your left arm to the side and up toward the ceiling. This will twist your body to the left as well. Look up toward your hand (8.5). Hold your breath in. *Asan Point.* Breathe out, bring your left hand down to the floor, and repeat the sequence on the opposite side.

4. Rest. Slowly lower your body to the floor on your stomach with forehead to the floor and arms stretched above your head. Rest until your breath returns to normal.

5. Baby Pose. Sit up on your heels and bend forward. If possible, rest your forehead on the floor, elbows bent to the sides (8.6). If your head does not reach the floor, just bend as far as possible with hips remaining on heels. Breathe out as you bend forward and hold the breath out. *Asan Point.* Breathe in and come up (note that in this sequence, you are using the Baby Pose as an asan, not as a rest pose), then rest. Lie on your back to rest in the Corpse Pose.

8.5

8.6

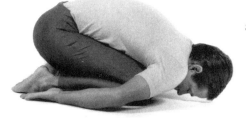

6. Cat Variation. This sequence is done with a strong, steady breath pattern. (a) Come up on hands and knees. Start by breathing in. Breathe out strongly as you round your back up and forward and bring your left knee to your forehead (8.7).

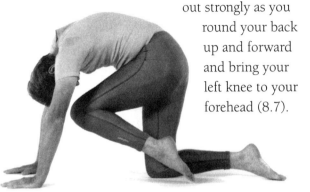

8.7

(b) Breathe in briefly as you release that position and breathe out again strongly as you straighten and lift your left leg in back, bend your elbows, and arch your back so your chin reaches toward the floor (8.8). Breathe in briefly as you release that position and breathe out as you go back to position 6(a) for the next repetition. Repeat three to six times on each side, slowly, then rest in the Baby Pose.

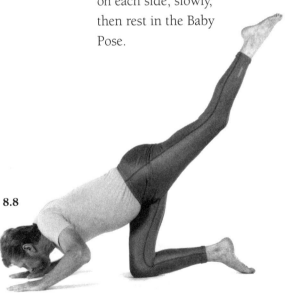

8.8

7. Plow Breath. (a) Sit up, swing your legs forward, and roll back, bringing your knees to your forehead (8.9). (b) Breathe in, hold a moment, then breathe out, extending your legs behind your head, carefully trying to touch your toes to the floor (8.10). Hold your breath out. *Asan Point.* (c) Breathe in and bend your knees back to your forehead, then roll forward to a cross-legged position, trying to place your forehead on the floor (8.11). Breathe naturally as you rest for about ten seconds. Repeat the entire sequence twice more. (Note: if you have a disk problem in your neck or upper back, do not do this exercise; substitute the Easy Bridge [see page 92].)

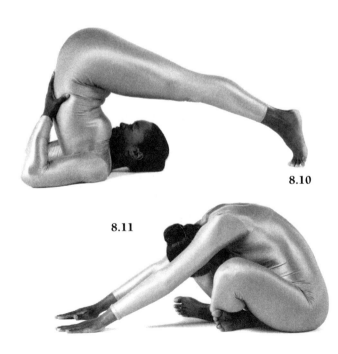

8.9

8.10

8.11

8. Rest on your back in the **Corpse Pose** (8.12) until breathing returns to normal (at least one minute).

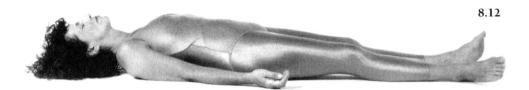

8.12

9. Big Sit-Up. (a) Raise your arms over your head on the floor and breathe out (8.13). (b) Breathe in as you lift both arms and legs, trying to

8.13

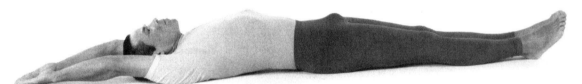

touch your toes without bending your knees (8.14). Hold your breath in. *Asan Point*. Breathe out and relax, bringing your arms back over your head on the floor as you lower your legs simultaneously. Repeat slowly three times, then rest in the Corpse Pose (8.12) until breathing returns to normal (at least one minute).

10. Alternate Big Sit-Up. Bring your right arm over your head on the floor and breathe out. Breathe in as you lift your right arm and left leg (opposites) and touch your toes, supporting yourself on your left elbow (8.15). Hold your breath in. *Asan Point*. Breathe out and lower. Repeat three times on each side, then rest in the Corpse Pose (8.12) until breath returns to normal.

8.14

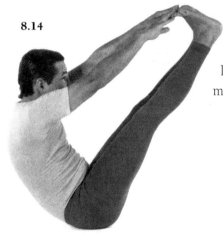

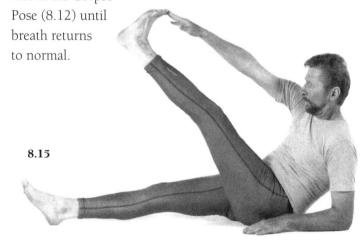

8.15

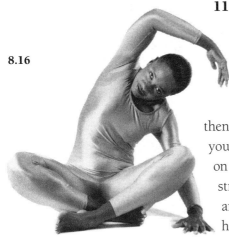

8.16

11. Side Stretch.
Sit up in a
comfortable
cross-legged
position.
Breathe in,
then breathe out as
you lean to the left
on your elbow and
stretch your right
arm up over your
head and toward
the left, stretching
the entire right side of your torso
(8.16). Hold the breath out. *Asan
Point.* Breathe in as you release and
repeat to the opposite side.

Balancing Both Halves of the Personality

The word *hatha* is made up of two
Sanskrit words: *ha* means sun, and
tha means moon. The sun and moon
are symbolic representations of the
right and left halves of the body and
mind; the aim of Hatha Yoga is to
balance the two sides so that they
can operate equally in order to create
a balanced, powerful individual.

The terms *Apollonian* and
Dionysian are often used to describe
these two opposite but harmonizing
aspects of the personality. In Greek
mythology, Apollo is the god of
music, poetry, prophecy, and medi-
cine; he governs the intellectual
aspects of life and art. Dionysus sym-

bolizes intoxication, instinct, emo-
tion, and passion. It is interesting to
note that in the Greek reference,
both of these qualities are represented by male figures. In Yogic literature, their counterparts are male
and female. In the Shaivite philosophy, the male and female are one
unit—the hermaphrodite. The following are some of the complemen-
tary qualities of this unit:

Apollonian	*Dionysian*
left nostril	right nostril
sun	moon
hot	cold
dry	wet
left brain	right brain
right side of body	left side of body
male	female
revealing	hiding
verbal	nonverbal
known	unknown
intellectual	spiritual

Usually one side dominates—but
it is never free of the response and
direction of the less-used side. For
instance, you use your left brain to
form words and sentences in order to
express a feeling, but your right
brain is where the impulse to the
feeling arises before you express it.
Someone who works all day with
numbers and logic, such as a computer programmer, is using mostly
the Apollonian side. Someone whose
work depends on emotions, such as
an actor, is using mostly the
Dionysian side.

If the two sides don't operate equally, you may feel out of balance: on days when you can easily balance your checkbook, you may find it difficult to talk about your emotions; on days when you are feeling very emotional, you may find it difficult to think logically. By balancing the two sides, Yoga gives you a choice: even though one side may be dominant, you can still use the other side. There is no need to be afraid of losing the strength of your dominant side by allowing the less dominant side to appear.

Most people experience one side of their nature operating most of the time; in many cases, they have been trained to view one side as more important than the other. For most people, this means that the Apollonian side is viewed as more productive, practical, and useful; the Dionysian side is hidden and frightening. By trying to ignore this hidden side, we lose a great deal of power in our personality. A person who uses primarily the Apollonian side will usually appear to be not very flexible; a person who uses primarily the Dionysian side will usually appear to be not strong or decisive. In order to practice Yoga successfully, one must begin to use both sides of the personality.

There is a scene in the striking film *Satyricon* that shows a beautiful hermaphrodite—a child that is half male and half female—hidden in a dark cave, guarded by wise men. The child lives in a golden cradle in half sleep, constantly bathed in pure water, all needs supplied in its ecstatic state. Robbers come in the night, thinking that they will obtain great magical powers by stealing the child for themselves. They ravage the cave, place the child in a rough cart, and start out across the desert with their prize. As the harsh sun beats down, the unprotected child dies.

In this story, the wet, dark, protected atmosphere of the cave was overcome by the hot, direct sun presence in the desert, destroying the delicate protection of the hermaphrodite. Similarly, in our own lives, the mysterious, unknown, magical, spiritual part of ourselves is often ignored. It may even be savaged by the demands of the opposite side, causing inflexibility, a split in the personality, and thus an inability to function as a powerful individual. This same scenario often happens in relationships. When heavy demands are made by one person, the other may seem to acquiesce, but a source of pain always remains, and problems eventually arise from this imbalance.

The term *Ha-tha* recognizes that the two parts exist simultaneously and that they are constantly trying to become more balanced. You will naturally improve that balance as you practice Yoga asans and breathing techniques, particularly the Alternate Nostril Breath (see Chapter 2). The two nostrils are described as sun and moon in Hatha, and by using the Alternate Nostril Breath, you can begin to balance your body and nervous system. When you practice this technique, you may experience how when the breath flows through one nostril, it heats the body, and when it flows through the other, it cools the body. This breath technique has been used in Yoga to be able to tolerate extreme temperatures happily.

There are two islands in Dal Lake in Kashmir. One is named Silver, and the other is named Gold. They represent the two nostrils and the two sides of the body. No one knows when they were first named, but my teacher Lakshmanjoo told me that they had those names during the lifetime of Abhinavagupta, the great teacher of Kashmir Shaivism.

Abhinavagupta's home in Kashmir was quite close to Lakshmanjoo's home, where I went for my class every day. Abhinavagupta lived in the tenth century and was a genius in representation of the ancient, esoteric practices of Yoga that existed in the Himalayas long before written history.

For many years, my teacher Rama (who was a contemporary of Lakshmanjoo) lived in the compound where Abhinavagupta had lived so long ago. Lakshmanjoo told me that he used to hear Rama in the night singing as he walked the hills; he said he used to warn Rama about the tigers that roamed in the hills in those days, but Rama went on singing in the night and he was never attacked.

9
The Powerful Individual

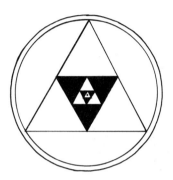

An aspect of desire

Many times when people begin to practice Yoga, they often cannot say what brought them to this decision. I used to begin every new class by asking each person: "Why are you here? What do you want from Yoga?" As I went around the room, very few people replied that they were there to practice and learn Yoga for its own sake. Most of them had other goals pressing: "My back hurts," "I can't sleep," "I'm depressed," "I want to improve my golf game," "I want to have a baby," and so on. (It is interesting to me that when the desired goal was reached, the person usually stopped practicing.) Every once in a while, however, the rare student emerges who is there simply to learn Yoga. I have been fortunate to meet a few such extraordinary people in my life.

Although students such as these are rare, there are many who are eager to use Yoga techniques to help them in various aspects of their lives. This is perfectly acceptable in Yoga, because Yoga makes no judgments about what people should believe or why they should practice. Yoga techniques are available for everyone to use for whatever goal they have in mind.

This adaptable quality of Yoga techniques will allow you to refine your daily routine to include techniques that will help you increase awareness and become a strong, powerful individual, able to move forward toward your personal goals.

This chapter includes three major sections. The first, "The Way You Live in the World," is a series of questionnaires that ask you about your attitudes, feelings, and habits in areas such as strength, flexibility, stress coping, concentration, self-image, and so on, plus your diet and other lifestyle matters. By answering these questions truthfully, you will get to know yourself better. If your score in any section is high, recommendations are provided for the techniques and routines in this book that will help you increase your personal power and awareness in those areas.

As in innumerable cups of water, many reflections of the sun are seen, but the substance is the same; similarly, individuals, like cups, are innumerable, but the vivifying spirit, like the sun, is one.

(Siva Samhita)

This is not a scientific test, but it has been systematically designed so that you will get a broader picture of your attitudes and behavior in several dimensions of everyday life. We consulted a clinical psychologist (who is also a Yoga student) to review the entire process and help with format and interpretation, and we used a cross-section of our own students to help shape the questions.

The second section, "The Shape You're In," has to do with your physical condition. By performing a series of prescribed movements, some in front of a mirror, you can judge your strength, limberness, and stamina for a variety of Yoga asans. Even though I do not emphasize physical culture above all else in Yoga, I do believe that it is important to practice Yoga asans for all-around fitness. Each section includes recommendations for exercises that will help correct areas of stiffness or weakness.

The third section is called "What Type of Student Are You?" In the 40-plus years that I have been teaching and observing students, I have noticed several distinct types. Sometimes people get stuck in a pattern of thought or behavior that evaporates when they become aware of it. Other times, it takes some extra effort to lift yourself out of a rut. Read all the different student types and see if you recognize yourself in any of them. Each description includes some recommendations for change if you so desire.

Section One: The Way You Live in the World

For each statement, circle the number that you believe best describes you. Score yourself within each section by adding the numbers circled. The *Recommendations* after each section suggest some techniques that may help if you score high in that area. Remember, this is not a scientific test, but merely a way to help you start learning more about yourself so you can use Yoga techniques more effectively.

DECISIVENESS

1. I weigh all aspects of a problem a very long time before making a decision.

   1 = never   2 = seldom
   3 = occasionally   4 = usually
   5 = always

2. After making a decision, I am confident I made the right choice.
   5 = never   4 = seldom
   3 = occasionally   2 = usually
   1 = always

3. I regret my decisions.
   1 = never   2 = seldom
   3 = occasionally   4 = usually
   5 = always

4. I do not have the energy to make decisions.
   1 = never   2 = seldom
   3 = occasionally   4 = usually
   5 = always

5. I think I am considered a decisive person.
   5 = never   4 = seldom
   3 = occasionally   2 = usually
   1 = always

6. I put off making decisions until the last minute.
   1 = never   2 = seldom
   3 = occasionally   4 = usually
   5 = always

Score: _____

Recommendations: If you scored high in this section (24 or above), you may benefit from using both the fantasy techniques described in Chapter 3. The "I Love You" Fantasy Technique will improve your self-confidence, and you may find it helpful to take an important decision or confrontation into one of the rooms in your fantasy hallway as a way to practice facing it. Practice the Emotional Stability Routine (Chapter 8) and the Sun Salutation (Chapter 4) at least four times a week. Do the Complete Breath (Chapter 2) every day.

EMOTIONAL STRENGTH

1. I feel overwhelmed by everything I have to do.
   1 = never   2 = seldom
   3 = occasionally   4 = usually
   5 = always

2. I feel that other people "walk all over me."
   1 = never   2 = seldom
   3 = occasionally   4 = usually
   5 = always

3. I have trouble getting what I want from salespeople.
   1 = never   2 = seldom
   3 = occasionally   4 = usually
   5 = always

4. It's easy for me to talk about how I am feeling.
   5 = never   4 = seldom
   3 = occasionally   2 = usually
   1 = always

5. I take good care of myself.
   5 = never   4 = seldom
   3 = occasionally   2 = usually
   1 = always

6. I am a good listener.
   5 = never   4 = seldom
   3 = occasionally   2 = usually
   1 = always

7. I feel that others don't understand me when I say something.
   1 = never   2 = seldom
   3 = occasionally   4 = usually
   5 = always

Score: _____

Recommendations: A high score in this section (28 or above) may indicate that you could benefit from working toward greater steadiness and awareness of your feelings. Practice the Emotional Stability Routine (Chapter 8) every day, and include the Cooling Breath (Chapter 2) to help you focus. Practice the "I Love You" Fantasy Technique to improve your self-image.

FLEXIBILITY

1. I enjoy surprises and being spontaneous.
   - 5 = never   4 = seldom
   - 3 = occasionally   2 = usually
   - 1 = always
2. I become upset when my regular daily schedule is disrupted.
   - 1 = never   2 = seldom
   - 3 = occasionally   4 = usually
   - 5 = always
3. I am aware of feeling angry much of the time.
   - 1 = never   2 = seldom
   - 3 = occasionally   4 = usually
   - 5 = always
4. I like going to new places (restaurants, shops, vacations, etc.).
   - 5 = never   4 = seldom
   - 3 = occasionally   2 = usually
   - 1 = always
5. I like to rearrange furniture and redecorate my surroundings.
   - 5 = never   4 = seldom
   - 3 = occasionally   2 = usually
   - 1 = always

Score: _____

Recommendations: If you scored high in this section (20 or above),

you may be expressing a pattern of rigidity that may hold you back from progress in advanced Yoga practice. Since emotional conditions are often expressed in the body, you may benefit from doing either the Flexibility Routine (Chapter 6) or the Emotional Stability Routine (Chapter 8) every day. Try to do your daily meditation with no expectations of the outcome. Practice the Alternate Nostril Breath (Chapter 2) daily to bring more balance into your personality. Try the "Hall of Space" Fantasy Technique (Chapter 3) with no expectations of what lies behind the doors to help you become more comfortable with the unknown.

ENERGY

1. I feel very tired during the day.
   - 1 = never   2 = seldom
   - 3 = occasionally   4 = usually
   - 5 = always
2. I find myself turning down invitations because I need to rest.
   - 1 = never   2 = seldom
   - 3 = occasionally   4 = usually
   - 5 = always
3. I wake in the morning feeling refreshed and ready for the day.
   - 5 = never   4 = seldom
   - 3 = occasionally   2 = usually
   - 1 = always
4. I feel "worn out" when I get home from work or school.
   - 1 = never   2 = seldom
   - 3 = occasionally   4 = usually
   - 5 = always

5. I have "above average" energy.
    5 = never   4 = seldom
    3 = occasionally   2 = usually
    1 = always

6. I depend on caffeine or other stimulants for energy.
    1 = never   2 = seldom
    3 = occasionally   4 = usually
    5 = always

7. I feel guilty about taking a nap.
    1 = never   2 = seldom
    3 = occasionally   4 = usually
    5 = always

8. I prefer to walk instead of drive when possible.
    5 = never   4 = seldom
    3 = occasionally   2 = usually
    1 = always

Score: _____

Recommendations: If you scored 32 or above in this section, you can begin to enjoy greater energy in your life by practicing the carefully designed Strength Routine (Chapter 5) and the Soft Bellows Breath (Chapter 2) every day along with the Sun Salutation and the Health Mantram (Chapter 4). If you can, add a few exercises from the Fatigue Routine (Chapter 4) each day into your routine as well. If your energy level remains low even after a week of this routine, check your diet to be sure you are getting enough protein, and check the status of your emotions. Emotional upset can be quite taxing; if you believe that you are not managing your emotions well, prac-

tice the Emotional Stability Routine (Chapter 8) for a week or two for extra support.

FEARFULNESS

1. I like taking risks.
    5 = never   4 = seldom
    3 = occasionally   2 = usually
    1 = always

2. I enjoy doing things I've never done before.
    5 = never   4 = seldom
    3 = occasionally   2 = usually
    1 = always

3. I enjoy meeting new people.
    5 = never   4 = seldom
    3 = occasionally   2 = usually
    1 = always

4. I consider myself a worrier.
    1 = never   2 = seldom
    3 = occasionally   4 = usually
    5 = always

5. I avoid confrontations whenever possible.
    1 = never   2 = seldom
    3 = occasionally   4 = usually
    5 = always

6. I enjoy going out to a play or movie alone.
    5 = never   4 = seldom
    3 = occasionally   2 = usually
    1 = always

Score: _____

Recommendations: Fearfulness can be greatly reduced by getting to know yourself better. If you scored 24 or above in this section, practice the "I Love You" Fantasy Technique (Chapter 3) every day to reduce anxiety. Use the Balance Routine (Chapter 7) and the Complete Breath (Chapter 2) to improve strength and steadiness of mind, and remove fear.

CONCENTRATION

1. I have trouble keeping my attention on one thing for more than a few minutes.

   1 = never   2 = seldom

   3 = occasionally   4 = usually

   5 = always

2. When I watch television, I'm a "channel surfer."

   1 = never   2 = seldom

   3 = occasionally   4 = usually

   5 = always

3. I like reading long magazine articles or books.

   5 = never   4 = seldom

   3 = occasionally   2 = usually

   1 = always

4. I enjoy taking on projects that involve lots of time and many details.

   5 = never   4 = seldom

   3 = occasionally   2 = usually

   1 = always

5. I enjoy working with numbers (e.g., bookkeeping, inventory, etc.).

   5 = never   4 = seldom

   3 = occasionally   2 = usually

   1 = always

6. I have a good memory.

   5 = never   4 = seldom

   3 = occasionally   2 = usually

   1 = always

7. I depend on my memory.

   5 = never   4 = seldom

   3 = occasionally   2 = usually

   1 = always

Score: _____

Recommendations: If your score is 28 or above, you may benefit from doing the Concentration and Balance Routines in Chapter 7 every day. Remember to use the Asan Point with each exercise to stop all thought momentarily; this allows the brain to rest from its usual chatter, and after this moment of silence, creative thought resumes in a new, refreshed way. Practice the Cooling Breath (Chapter 2) before your daily meditation.

DIET AND HEALTH

1. I take vitamins or other nutritional supplements daily.

   5 = never   4 = seldom

   3 = occasionally   2 = usually

   1 = always

2. I eat breakfast every day.

   5 = never   4 = seldom

   3 = occasionally   2 = usually

   1 = always

3. I have regular medical checkups.

   5 = never   4 = seldom

   3 = occasionally   2 = usually

   1 = always

4. I eat lunch "on the run."

   1 = never   2 = seldom

   3 = occasionally   4 = usually

   5 = always

5. I buy a lot of convenience foods.
   1 = never   2 = seldom
   3 = occasionally   4 = usually
   5 = always

6. I exercise regularly (in addition to Yoga).
   5 = never   4 = seldom
   3 = occasionally   2 = usually
   1 = always

7. My refrigerator always contains fresh produce and milk.
   5 = never   4 = seldom
   3 = occasionally   2 = usually
   1 = always

8. I try every new diet or exercise program that comes along.
   1 = never   2 = seldom
   3 = occasionally   4 = usually
   5 = always

9. My weight is within the recommended range for my height and age.
   5 = never   4 = seldom
   3 = occasionally   2 = usually
   1 = always

Score: _____

Recommendations: A high score in this section is 36 or above. Most students are aware that diet is important, but even advanced students often fail to ensure that their diet is complete every day. The most common excuse is, "I don't have time right now." I have noticed that people who are too busy to take care of their nutrition usually have poor self-esteem and are often very driven and competitive. This is a stressful condition that needs the utmost support from a balanced diet. The "I Love You" Fantasy Technique (Chapter 3) will help greatly to enhance and soften your image of yourself. Add the Health Mantram, the Sun Salutation, and the Fatigue Routine (all in Chapter 4) to your daily routine as well.

LIFESTYLE AND SCHEDULE

1. My job requires long hours of sitting or standing.
   1 = never   2 = seldom
   3 = occasionally   4 = usually
   5 = always

2. I spend several hours a day working at a computer terminal.
   1 = never   2 = seldom
   3 = occasionally   4 = usually
   5 = always

3. I have children under age eighteen at home.
   1 = none   2 = one
   3 = two   4 = three
   5 = more than three

4. My normal workday is longer than eight hours.
   1 = never   2 = seldom
   3 = occasionally   4 = usually
   5 = always

5. I get along with my coworkers.
   5 = never   4 = seldom
   3 = occasionally   2 = usually
   1 = always

6. I have time for hobbies and other things I do for enjoyment.
   5 = never   4 = seldom
   3 = occasionally   2 = usually
   1 = always

7. I worry about not doing my work perfectly.

 1 = never   2 = seldom
 3 = occasionally   4 = usually
 5 = always

8. I find myself working, taking calls from work, or thinking about work a lot even when I'm at home.

 1 = never   2 = seldom
 3 = occasionally   4 = usually
 5 = always

Score: _____

Recommendations: If you scored 32 or above in this section, you may be under a great deal of stress due to an extremely busy lifestyle. Your answers to the questions in this section should clearly show you what you are doing to yourself in your life and what your priorities are. Now is the time to evaluate your schedule and see if it is giving you what you really want.

If you are feeling imprisoned by your lifestyle, Yoga can free you. You can learn to make choices according to what you really want, instead of what you feel you *ought* to do. If you feel trapped, make a conscious effort to free yourself. Don't go on suffering in silence. Many people are surprised to find out that no one really cares about your suffering except you, and you are the only one who can do anything to change it.

Alternate the Balance Routine (Chapter 7) with the Emotional Stability Routine (Chapter 8). Using the "I Love You" Fantasy Technique (Chapter 3) before meditation will be very helpful. Use the "Hall of Space" Fantasy Technique (Chapter 3) to design a lifestyle and schedule you will really enjoy. Learn to say "no" gently and happily. I have observed that people who never say no are usually angry at everyone. This can be corrected with a committed daily practice of the techniques described above.

SELF-IMAGE

1. I feel good about how I look.

 5 = never   4 = seldom
 3 = occasionally   2 = usually
 1 = always

2. I feel good about how my life is going.

 5 = never   4 = seldom
 3 = occasionally   2 = usually
 1 = always

3. I am on a diet.

 1 = never   2 = seldom
 3 = occasionally   4 = usually
 5 = always

4. I avoid shopping for new clothes.

 1 = never   2 = seldom
 3 = occasionally   4 = usually
 5 = always

5. I have "ugly fits."

 1 = never   2 = seldom
 3 = occasionally   4 = usually
 5 = always

6. I enjoy changing my appearance.
   5 = never   4 = seldom
   3 = occasionally   2 = usually
   1 = always

7. I feel better about myself when I complete a job successfully.
   5 = never   4 = seldom
   3 = occasionally   2 = usually
   1 = always

Score: _____

Recommendations: A high score in this section is 28 or above. Most of us have a fantasy picture of what we think we are supposed to be; when you begin to pay attention to your self-image, you gain the important knowledge of who you really are. The "I Love You" Fantasy Technique (Chapter 3) will allow you to become compassionate and tender toward yourself. This makes for a much easier adjustment to the image you want to be, as opposed to the harsh, unrealistic goals that many people whip themselves with and that are usually impossible to attain. Practice the Strength Routine (Chapter 5) and the Fatigue Routine (Chapter 4), alternating days if you wish, and do several repetitions of Complete Breath (Chapter 2) before meditation.

STRESS

1. I hold grudges.
   1 = never   2 = seldom
   3 = occasionally   4 = usually
   5 = always

2. I find myself "sailing through" everyday obstacles such as traffic delays, bad weather, demands from family and work, etc.
   5 = never   4 = seldom
   3 = occasionally   2 = usually
   1 = always

3. I experience physical symptoms such as rapid heartbeat, stomach upset, headache, back pain, frequent sighing (not due to a known illness).
   1 = never   2 = seldom
   3 = occasionally   4 = usually
   5 = always

4. I can easily get to sleep and stay asleep.
   5 = never   4 = seldom
   3 = occasionally   2 = usually
   1 = always

5. I feel anxious without knowing why.
   1 = never   2 = seldom
   3 = occasionally   4 = usually
   5 = always

6. I eat a balanced, healthy diet, even when I'm upset.
   5 = never   4 = seldom
   3 = occasionally   2 = usually
   1 = always

7. I feel depressed or "blue."
   1 = never   2 = seldom
   3 = occasionally   4 = usually
   5 = always

8. I worry a lot about things I am unable to control (war, famine, the homeless, etc.).
   1 = never   2 = seldom
   3 = occasionally   4 = usually
   5 = always

9. I feel responsible for other people's actions.
    1 = never   2 = seldom
    3 = occasionally 4 = usually
    5 = always

Score: _____

Recommendations: Stress seems to be a way of life in the United States. You can love it or you can hate it; either way it takes a toll on the body and emotions. If you scored high in this section (36 or above), you will need to keep a careful watch on yourself to avoid becoming ill. Check your diet every day. Use the Fatigue Routine (Chapter 4) or the Strength Routine (Chapter 5) every day, depending on your time schedule. The ideal would be to alternate them. Before you do any practices for the day, repeat the Health Mantram (Chapter 4), and do three repetitions of the Rising Breath (Chapter 2) just before meditation.

Practice these techniques as a whole "package." You will not get the same results by doing just part of it. If you have severe time constraints on some days, do fewer asans (at least three exercises, repeated three times) but do not cut your breathing or meditation times. Make your daily effort a complete unit.

ROMANCE AND FRIENDSHIP

1. I feel lonely.
    1 = never   2 = seldom
    3 = occasionally 4 = usually
    5 = always

2. I have recently (in the past year) experienced a breakup of a love affair.
    5 = yes   1 = no

3. I have good friends.
    5 = none   4 = one
    3 = a few   2 = three to
    1 = many   five

4. I have recently lost a loved one or a very good friend.
    5 = yes (more than one in the past year)
    4 = yes (one in the past year)
    3 = yes (one in the past two years)
    2 = yes (one in the past five years)
    1 = no

5. I feel lots of support around me when I'm going through a crisis.
    5 = never   4 = seldom
    3 = occasionally 2 = usually
    1 = always

6. I am a jealous person.
    1 = never   2 = seldom
    3 = occasionally 4 = usually
    5 = always

7. I feel that the perfect relationship would solve all my problems.
    1 = never   2 = seldom
    3 = occasionally 4 = usually
    5 = always

8. I am happiest when I'm with other people.
    5 = never   4 = seldom
    3 = occasionally 2 = usually
    1 = always

Score: _____

Recommendations: The beautiful qualities of romance and friendship cannot exist in a climate of competition and demand. The phrase "you need to bring something to the table" is apt when talking about relationships of any kind. Most people have an unconscious expectation that everyone whom they love or are friends with will fix everything for them. It is such unspoken feelings that destroy the tender qualities of a relationship.

If you scored 32 or above in this section, you may want to explore ways to bring more balance to your relationships, giving them a better chance to endure. Practice the "I Love You" Fantasy Technique (Chapter 3) every day. Find out if you love yourself or if you don't—and if you're expecting everyone else to do it for you. People who learn to love themselves become much less demanding or critical, because it becomes painful to be so. Compassion flows as you relax into your breath exercises and meditation. Compassion is infectious; it starts with yourself and spreads to others.

MYSTICAL QUALITIES

1. I have had dreams about mythical figures or spiritual leaders.
   5 = never   4 = seldom
   3 = occasionally   2 = usually
   1 = always

2. I feel that an unseen force or quality is guiding my life.
   5 = never   4 = seldom
   3 = occasionally   2 = usually
   1 = always

3. I like to think about what the concept of God means to me.
   5 = never   4 = seldom
   3 = occasionally   2 = usually
   1 = always

4. I wonder about what happens after death.
   5 = never   4 = seldom
   3 = occasionally   2 = usually
   1 = always

5. I enjoy talking to others about philosophical or spiritual issues.
   5 = never   4 = seldom
   3 = occasionally   2 = usually
   1 = always

6. I enjoy reading about mythology, religion, philosophy, mysticism, or psychology.
   5 = never   4 = seldom
   3 = occasionally   2 = usually
   1 = always

7. I have premonitions about things.
   5 = never   4 = seldom
   3 = occasionally   2 = usually
   1 = always

Score: _____

Recommendations: Mystical qualities are the frosting on the cake of personality. As we plod along in our everyday lives, doing what we must do to survive, the delightful, surprising entry of spontaneous mystical thought is like a burst of hopeful sunshine. For most of us, these eruptions have been silenced in early childhood. "Stop dreaming and get to work!" is the phrase we often hear in our heads when a daydream or fantasy enchants us, even as adults. We are taught to believe that these entries into the mystical part of ourselves are not useful or productive. Yoga, on the other hand, states that unless the flow from the unconscious is unrestricted and easily available, the person will suffer from severe stress. In fact, Yogic philosophy goes so far as to assert that the mystical side of our nature is our real support. The body cannot become truly healthy or happy without conscious effort to recognize it, and there can be no real progress or success without it. Our mystical nature is the real source of intuition and creativity. You cannot be a person of real depth without training to use this tremendous source of power that lies within you.

If you scored 28 or above in this section, perhaps you would like to experiment with "unblocking" your mystical nature. Practice the "Hall of Space" Fantasy Technique (Chapter 3) daily, and write down your experiences and dialogue with the unconscious part of yourself. Keep track of when you hear your intuitive voice speak and have the courage to follow its directions—and remember also what happens when that voice is denied.

To help encourage your mystical side to emerge, do the Emotional Stability Routine (Chapter 8) faithfully several times a week, and even when you change to another routine, add a few exercises from the Emotional Stability Routine. Daily practice of the Alternate Nostril Breath (Chapter 2) will balance both sides of your person-

ality. Meditate every day, stopping all thought. Be comfortable not knowing.

Section Two: The Shape You're In

PHYSICAL STRENGTH AND LIMBERNESS

The following exercises will help you assess your physical condition and suggest ways in which to improve strength or limberness. Many exercises have more than one function. Remember that these are assessment tools only; when you practice Yoga exercises, do not force your body to exceed its limitations. Strength and limberness are not ends in themselves, but means to achieve better health. Do a full warm-up routine (see Chapter 2) before anything else. Wear a leotard or other formfitting clothing. Have a full-length mirror nearby if possible.

Limberness—Spine and Back of Legs

Stand sideways in front of a full-length mirror. Bend forward from the waist, keeping your knees straight but not locked, and let your arms and hands dangle (9.1). Hang for several seconds to let your muscles relax to their fullest extent. Do your fingers touch the floor? When you look in the mirror, is your back bent evenly or is there a section that seems straighter?

Now sit with legs outstretched. Reach forward as far as you can, keeping your knees straight and feet flexed toward your face (9.3). Do your hands reach to your knees? Calves? Ankles? Feet? Beyond your toes?

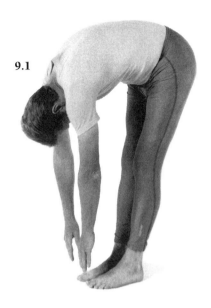

9.1

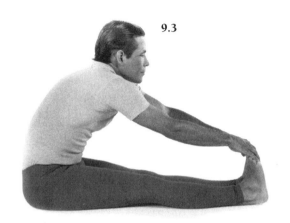

9.3

Now lie on your stomach with your forehead on the floor. Place your hands palms down next to your shoulders and keep your feet together. Breathe in as you curl your head back, eyes looking up into your forehead, and continue curling your back, keeping your hipbones on the floor (9.2). When you look up as far as you can, are you looking at the ceiling or the wall? Is there discomfort in your lower back that is relieved when you separate your feet? Are your arms straight or bent?

Recommendations: To stretch and limber your spinal column in both directions, practice exercises such as the Standing and Seated Sun Poses (Chapter 6), the Sun Salutation (Chapter 4), the Cobra V-Raise (Chapter 5), the Cobra Pose (Chapter 7), the Bow Variation (Chapter 7), the Bow Pose (Chapter 5), the Wheel (Chapter 6), and the Pigeon Pose (Chapter 4).

Balance

Stare at one spot on the wall in front of you and balance on one foot. Lift your other foot in front of you and circle your ankle several times in each direction (9.4). Time yourself, and stop when you feel

9.2

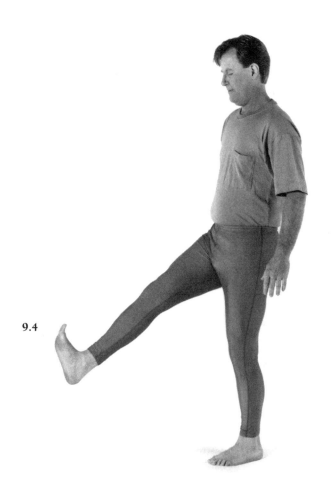

9.4

Limberness—Knee Joint

Can you easily sit on your feet with knees together without strain on your knees?

Sit cross-legged on the floor on a cushion or two with one heel drawn in toward your groin and the other foot on the floor directly in front of it (9.5). Do your knees touch the floor?

Recommendations: Practice the Fatigue Routine (Chapter 4) at least four times a week to limber the hips and knees. When you change to other routines, always include the Hero Pose, the Alternate Seated Sun Pose, the "Telephone" Pose, and the Spine Twist (all in Chapter 6). Sit cross-legged as often as you can: for instance, while watching television or reading. If you spend a lot of time sitting in an office chair, try drawing one foot up on the inside of the other thigh as often as possible, alternating sides.

your body starting to shake. Do the same on the other foot.

Recommendations: To improve balance and coordination, practice the Balance Routine (Chapter 7) at least four times a week. Practice balancing on one foot at other times of the day, such as when talking on the phone or waiting in line. Sometimes chronically poor balance indicates a weak nervous system. Check your diet: are you getting enough protein and B vitamins? Are you getting enough rest? Are you allowing time for relaxation during the day?

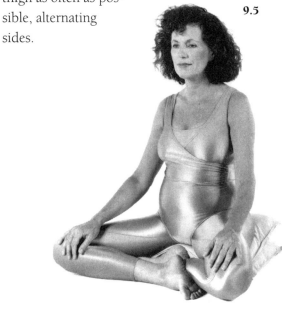

9.5

Limberness—Thighs

9.6

Sit on your feet with knees together. Lean back on your elbows as far as you can without strain, until you feel the muscles in your thighs stretched just to the point *before* they become uncomfortable (9.6). How far back can you go?

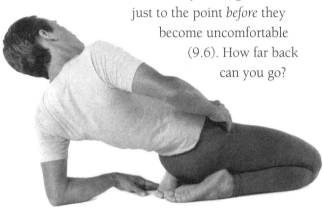

Sit with legs apart as far as possible. Reach forward with both hands (9.7). How far can you go?

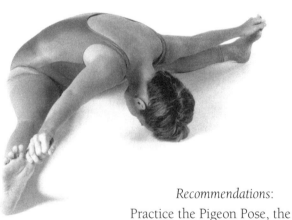

Recommendations: Practice the Pigeon Pose, the **9.7** Fish Pose, the Camel Pose (Chapter 4), and the Bow Variation (Chapter 7) to stretch the front of the thigh. To work on the inner thigh area, practice the Tortoise Stretch and Alternate Seated Sun Pose (both in Chapter 6) and the Lunge Series (Chapter 5).

Back Strength

Sit on the floor cross-legged, with your usual pillow support under your hips. How long can you sit before your back begins to slump?

Recommendations: To strengthen your back, sit without a back support as often as you can. In your exercise routine, include the Back Strengthener Series and the T Pose and variations (Chapter 5), the Arm and Leg Balance (Chapter 7), the Cobra V-Raise (Chapter 5), and the Locust Pose (Chapter 7).

Limberness—Upper and Lower Back

In a standing position, reach back with both arms straight. Can you touch your hands together? Clasp your hands? Lock your elbows so your shoulder blades are squeezed together (9.8)?

9.8

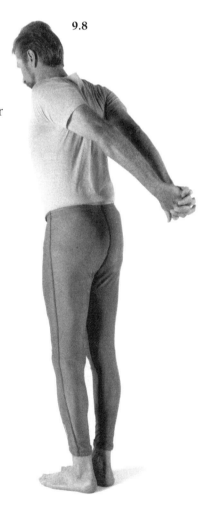

Lie on the floor on your back. Lift your arms overhead and straighten them (9.9). Do your shoulders touch the floor?

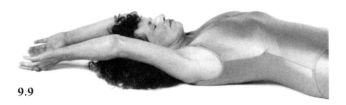

9.9

Lie on your stomach with arms out to each side and forehead on the floor. Bend your left leg so the knee is parallel to your hip. Turn your feet inward and try to touch both heels to the floor without strain (9.10). Repeat on the other side. How far can you go?

Recommendations: The first two tests will show you the beginnings of a rounded or hunched upper back. To correct this problem, practice the Full Bend Variation (Chapter 2), the Pigeon Pose Variation (Chapter 5), and the Bow Variation (Chapter 7). The Side Triangle (Chapter 5), the Twisting Triangle (Chapter 5), the

Camel Pose (Chapter 4), the Cobra Pose (Chapter 7), and the Bow Pose (Chapter 5) will also help loosen the upper torso. The third test shows a stiffness in the lower back. To help loosen it, practice the Standing and Seated Sun Poses and Alternate Seated Sun Pose and the Tortoise Stretch (Chapter 6), the Camel and Pigeon Poses (Chapter 4), the Cobra Pose, and the Bow Variation (both in Chapter 7).

Section Three: What Type of Student Are You?

THE SHOPPER

"Shopper" students are not ready to make a commitment to any particular fitness program. Probably they do not practice Yoga daily because their schedule is full of many other types of fitness/holistic practices besides Yoga, such as Tai Chi, aerobics, weights, etc. They are unsure of their personal goals.

Recommendations: If you try one program alone for at least three months, instead of trying several things at once, you'll have a clearer picture of whether you

9.10

like it, what benefits it gives you, and whether you want to continue.

THE HELPLESS STUDENT

"Helpless" students have no idea why Yoga has entered their life, but they feel a drive to do it, so they keep on practicing despite a lack of specific goals.

Comments: Often Yoga will appear in a person's life without any warning, as it did to me in my early twenties. I suppose I was lucky in that I had no preconceptions about what Yoga was or what I might experience. When you are free from expectations, you won't be limited in the results. Yoga changes a person from being a victim to being a strong individual with choices. You will have to decide if you enjoy being helpless. Just making this decision begins to remove you from the prison of helplessness.

THE OVERACHIEVER

Some people plunge into Yoga with very intense effort, thinking that they can know everything in a short time and then move on. They take on too much self-discipline too quickly, and become overloaded and stressed—they may even burn out and stop practicing altogether.

Recommendations: I must first ask: What do you plan to move on to? If you are a perfectionist, you may become frustrated by this over-

achieving style of practice. You cannot force Yoga onto yourself or anyone else. After many years of practice, I have come to realize that Yoga moves at its own pace. Try to ease up on yourself a little. Set a minimum time to practice every day—even just three exercises and a few minutes of meditation will be enough to keep the momentum of daily practice going—and don't be hard on yourself if you are unable to do more than the minimum on some days. Learn to enjoy the feelings of the present moment instead of always setting impossibly high standards for yourself. Use your Yoga practice as a daily input of support toward having the strength to do what you want to do happily.

THE ESCAPIST

This student usually embraces Yoga because it is so different from his or her normal life and often seems more rewarding. This student looks to Yoga for solutions to all of life's problems and may "lean" on Yoga and Yoga teachers, expecting them to provide not only health and well-being, but also comradeship, counseling, and sometimes even a religious-type belief system. This person then often becomes disillusioned and depressed when Yoga class doesn't provide all the answers.

Recommendations: Someone who is practicing Yoga to escape from an unhappy life must eventually face the difficult truth that Yoga does not solve life's problems; it simply teaches you how to become stronger and healthier and more aware so that you can solve your own problems. Trying to run away from life achieves nothing. My great teacher Lakshmanjoo said that real detachment comes from attachment; in other words, take care of the things on your mind first—then you can concentrate on Yoga. If you go off to a cave to meditate, but you spend your time thinking about what you have left behind, you have not really left it behind at all! By paying attention to what most concerns you, you will finish those matters; then you can meditate more easily. This means you must learn to keep your word; either take care of the things that are troubling you or dismiss them.

THE COMPETENT STUDENT

This person works at Yoga steadily and regularly, meticulously following all instructions and suggestions. This student is generally fairly healthy and is practicing Yoga with the goal of maintaining health and well-being and, possibly, the additional goal of searching for greater meaning in life.

Recommendations: The *Bhagavad Gita* says that four types of people practice Yoga: the sufferer, the seeker for knowledge, the seeker for worldly goods, and the wise. I have seen many people practice Yoga with some particular goal in mind, whether conscious or not. When the goal is achieved, the person stops practicing. There is nothing wrong with this. I believe that the practice of Yoga in our lives comes and goes on its own time schedule. Whatever your reason for practicing, Yoga can present you with the opportunity to find out more about yourself. There is constant, steady action of uniting your inner self to your social, public, outer self. The product that emerges—you as a whole person—will surprise you.

THE FOLLOWER

This student wants to belong to a group, finding safety and meaning in letting others tell him or her what to do. This person is very eager to do everything right and does not trust his or her own judgment or common sense.

Recommendations: People with this desire often become frustrated because true teachers do not allow students to turn them into a religious figure of some sort or build a "personality cult" around them. Yoga may, of course, be learned in a group class, and sharing experiences, ideas, and questions with other students is helpful, but in the final analysis, Yoga must be practiced alone. The role of the teacher is to teach the techniques of Yoga correctly and guide students in interpreting their experiences, but the student is eventually urged to strong independence.

THE TRAPPED STUDENT

People who feel trapped are always tormented by the idea that they would be better off doing something else. They try one thing after another, but the feeling remains. Their efforts are always somewhat watered down, making it difficult for them to progress. Sometimes there is a tendency to blame others for their predicament.

Recommendations: This person's unhappiness is usually caused by focusing on the future or the past. The best remedy for this trapped feeling is concentration on the present moment and being able to deal with it. A greater awareness of how to do this will emerge as you do your Yoga techniques daily. On difficult days you can cut your daily practice to the minimum, but try to do everything with utmost concentration. Do at least three exercises every day and pay attention to how they feel, if you can. Do at least three repetitions of Complete Breath, and meditate for a minimum of ten minutes. Meditation will rest your mind from the tenacious inner thought that recurs and is so tiring. This continual break from one train of thought that bothers you will weaken it and eventually free you.

Take time every week to consider how you are feeling compared to last week, last month, and six months ago. Write some notes to yourself and keep them in a conspicuous place—posted on your refrigerator, for instance—and check them every day. Replace them weekly with new observations.

THE REBOUND STUDENT

"Rebound" students dive into Yoga practice with great zeal, adopting every restrictive discipline that they mistakenly believe Yoga requires, such as strict celibacy, a limited diet, and hours of disciplined practice every day. Naturally, they are unable to sustain such restraint all at once, and after a while they leave Yoga entirely and go back to their former lifestyle, often overcompensating with an excess of sex, drugs, alcohol, or food. If they return to Yoga, it is with great guilt and a desire to punish themselves with even more restrictive practices, repeating the cycle over again.

Recommendations: Many people approach Yoga with a religious attitude, seeing Yoga as a substitute for the religious tradition in which they were raised and transferring the "shalt nots" from childhood lessons. Yoga is not religion, and carries no universal moralistic proscriptions. In fact, one of the most important concepts is nonviolence, starting with not being harmful to oneself. Forcing yourself to adhere to rigid rules is a form of self-violence. Advanced Yoga students do usually change their diet and practice short periods of celibacy, but these are always individual decisions made when the student is ready for the extra discipline and with the close observation of an excellent teacher who has been through this experience.

THE FENCE RIDER

"Fence Rider" students won't decide where to put their energy; they won't quite commit their efforts to regular, attentive Yoga practice—or anything else. They fear failure, letdown, nonacceptance, incompetence, and losing control, yet they are inviting these things by being indecisive. They don't trust their teachers or themselves, so their half-efforts produce disappointing results. They are never strong individuals.

Recommendations: These students have no clear point of judgment to decide what to do. On the surface, it appears as if they do not know what they want; actually they do, but they don't want to admit it. If you find yourself "on the fence" in life, you will need to pay careful attention to the ethical guidelines of Yoga. You will have to take responsibility for yourself. Be brave! Don't run from your feelings. Talk to yourself honestly. To help you learn to identify your feelings, ask yourself questions like these:

- What's going on right now?
- Am I feeling miserable or in pain? If so, where does it hurt? How painful is it?

- Am I feeling mean? Angry? Sad? Bored? Hungry? Ugly? Sexy? Excited? Fearful? Anxious? Lonely?
- Am I feeling a reaction to something someone said to me?
- Am I feeling a burden?
- Will eating make me feel better? Worse?
- Do I need to rest?
- Am I anxious about a relationship?
- Do I feel like my efforts are wasted?
- Do I want to take responsibility for myself?

Usually, all these problems can be clarified by simply adhering to the ethical code of Yoga. You will find immediate relief by applying this code to anything that is upsetting you. Review the ten ethical guidelines of Yoga: nonviolence; truthfulness; refraining from stealing, casual sex, and hoarding; purity; contentment; tolerance; study; and remembrance. Ask yourself if you have moved away from any of these. For instance, are you being violent to yourself in any way? Have you kept your word to yourself? Are you trying to "own" something that cannot be owned? Can you remember the larger context? Have you practiced being content in the present moment? Have you considered taking responsibility for your own actions?

When you become accustomed to this practice, you will have an immediate cure on hand for upset or indecision. Confusion leaves as soon as it is measured against these fundamental ethics.

The Kundalini Experience

The word *kundalini* is much used in the United States these days, but very few people use the word correctly. The word is generally used in reference to a movement of energy up the spinal column that changes one's state of consciousness—at first, usually, in temporary flashes of insight, and later in states of awareness that gradually become more permanent. Those who practice Yoga intensively usually experience some movement of the force of kundalini.

My first experience of kundalini occurred the first time I sat in meditation with my great teacher, Rama. He had come to the United States at the invitation of a group of people who invited me to come along to meet him because they had heard of my interest in Yoga. There was a wonderful welcome for him when he got off the plane—a beautiful brown man looking like a prizefighter in a Kashmiri bathrobe. I just observed. I didn't say anything. I had been practicing Yoga for over ten years by then, but I had never had a chance to see a master up close. We drove back to someone's home for a reception in Rama's honor, and after the hospital-

ity of food and drink was provided, someone asked if Rama would sit in meditation with us for a little while.

We all gathered in a large living room. The people who were responsible for the affair were sitting in all the chairs and couches and there was nothing left for me to sit on but a piano bench. It was a little high for me; my feet were dangling. Rama said, "Now we will meditate a few moments." I had never meditated with anyone but myself. Rama began to sing the mantram *Om*. Suddenly some force shot up the back of my neck and threw me off the piano bench into the wall. I lay on the floor like an idiot, then made my way back to the piano bench, tears running down my face, totally humiliated by what had happened to me. Everyone else in the room was pretending to meditate. As I crawled back up on the piano bench, Rama looked right at me and said, "Well, I see the channels are open." And those are the only words he ever said about it.

From that day on I began to discover the power of kundalini. Eventually, I discovered that kundalini really, in the abstract sense, is nothing but a love affair with oneself. When two forces meet inside you, the experience is like sexual bliss but much more intense.

According to Yogic thought, kundalini lies asleep in everyone and can be awakened by specific training. People spend days or years trying to awaken this force in themselves— often in dangerous ways, such as by practicing violent breathing exercises or banging the end of their spine repeatedly on the floor, both of which can be extremely harmful. The way Rama described it to me, the body has two nervous systems—one that is seen and one that is unseen. The unseen system is a psychic nervous system that can be awakened with training that includes periods of celibacy and intense attention to diet. However, the kundalini experience cannot be forced to occur; its timing depends on many things, including your innermost desires and tendencies—things you may not even be aware of.

The first sign of the kundalini experience is a slight tickling around the hips in the back as you sit for meditation. You feel a slight warmth, and almost a kind of crawling sensation of something moving up the spine. Some people may not feel anything at all but may experience changes in perception or awareness as Yoga activates this second, subtle, nervous system.

When this experience of kundalini begins to happen, you must be extremely careful of yourself. You need to give yourself full, loving support. You must realize that awakening this extraordinary extra-nervous system in yourself requires that you take great care to eat a healthy vegetarian diet, get enough rest, and behave ethically; these are the essential habits that will sustain you through the experience. Without these supports, you risk overload and injury.

Another important support in this awakening experience is silence. Some time after I met Rama, I went back to India with him for advanced training. We lived in a primitive camp near the Ganges River in Haridwar. Rama imposed a long vow of silence on me, which served both as a discipline and a protection while this kundalini experience was coming on. Because of this silent time, I became extremely observant.

One thing I realized was that I had been living my life on only half of my personal power. The real union that comes when both nervous systems are operating in the brain is one of tremendous force. You are very lucky if you have a teacher nearby to support you during that time. However, if the experience is true and real, the teacher comes from within.

Kundalini is often given the name of a goddess—a goddess so in love with the state of consciousness called *Shiva* that she climbs and climbs, reaching for that sexual union in the brain. The male and female parts of the individual then become united; the result is that personal power becomes enormous. You recognize that love exists within yourself, not dependent on anything or anybody else. From that time on, all feeling of separateness disappears.

How to Choose a Yoga Teacher

This book has been written in a way that will allow you to begin a safe, rewarding practice of Yoga in your own home. If you do decide to try to find a Yoga class in your area, however, here are some guidelines to help you choose the most competent teacher.

There has never been any national or international certification program for Yoga teachers, and I doubt if there ever will be such a program because of the traditional nature of Yoga instruction. For many thousands of years, Yoga was transmitted from teacher to student on a one-to-one basis; only comparatively recently has Yoga been offered in a group class format. Advanced practice of Yoga still is best undertaken on a one-to-one basis, if you are lucky enough to find a competent teacher who is willing to teach you. Teaching Yoga is never a hobby or a sideline undertaken by someone who reads a couple of books and decides to become a Yoga teacher; he or she must be under the constant supervision of his or her personal Yoga teacher.

This relationship between teacher and student is taken very seriously by both parties and is never entered into lightly. I am highly amused by people who describe their teacher as their guru without the teacher's con-

sent. First of all, a teacher never describes himself or herself as a guru; this word is properly used only by the student. A guru relationship must be acknowledged by both parties and is based on a much deeper relationship than is comprehended by most Westerners. In Yoga treatises, one reads that this relationship is considered to continue even after death.

People are constantly asking me to recommend teachers in their area. Because of my belief in the strict training required for the teaching of Yoga, I have made it a policy never to recommend a teacher unless I have personally trained the person. This does not mean that there are no competent teachers available; you may just have to search a little harder. I cannot take responsibility for other people's teaching. There is an old saying: "When the student is ready, the teacher appears." However, it is only fair to add that the next verse reads, "One gets the teacher one deserves." This book will enable you to safely progress into intensive Yoga practice until you meet the teacher who is right for you.

In the following paragraphs, I have outlined what I believe are the minimum requirements for a competent teacher of Yoga.

1. *Daily practice of Yoga exercise, breathing, and meditation.* No one can make progress in Yoga without a serious commitment to daily practice.

A teacher *must* have this support in order to build the solid foundation of experience that is required before he or she can show others how to achieve that experience; daily practice is also needed to maintain the strength and health necessary for the extra demands of teaching.

2. *Regular contact with a teacher.* No teacher can work effectively in a vacuum, and no one becomes so advanced that he or she does not need the guidance and support of his or her own teacher.

3. *Study of the important Yoga texts.* Study is one of the five observances that are part of the essential eight "limbs" of Yoga practice (see 4, below). A teacher needs to have an intensive background of study that includes Patanjali's *Yoga Sutras*, the *Hatha Yoga Pradipika*, the *Bhagavad Gita*, and all world philosophies, at the very least.

4. *Ethical behavior.* The five *yamas* (meaning *restraints*: nonviolence, truthfulness, nonstealing, periods of celibacy, nonhoarding) and the five *niyamas* (meaning *observances*: purity, contentment, tolerance, study, remembrance) are the first two limbs in Patanjali's system of classical Yoga (called *Ashtanga Yoga*). The remaining six limbs are: (1) physical exercises (*asana*), (2) breathing techniques (*pranayama*), (3) withdrawal of the mind from the senses "as a turtle draws in its limbs" (*pratyahara*), (4) concentration, defined as selec-tive and voluntary dishabituation (*dharana*), (5) meditation (*dhyana*), and (6) absorption, or ultimate union with the self (*samadhi*). My teacher Lakshmanjoo once said that, like a child developing in the womb whose limbs grow all at once, rather than one by one, these eight limbs must be developed simultaneously.

The ethical guidelines of the yamas and niyamas are a part of Yoga practice not for moralistic reasons but because they support and protect the student during the unfolding of personal experience in meditation. A teacher needs this support and protection for the same reasons, as well as to help reduce the interference of personal ego in the teaching process.

An ethical Yoga teacher conducts classes in a responsible, safe, and aware manner; organizes classes that are not too large for each student to receive individual attention; and never pushes students beyond their limitations. Sexual involvement with students is absolutely prohibited.

5. *A healthy vegetarian diet.* Although you do not need to be a vegetarian to *practice* Yoga, a Yoga teacher must conform to different standards. Someone who is taking responsibility for teaching others how to use Yoga meditation techniques must have the steadiness and nonviolent attitude that can only be attained through a vegetarian diet. See Chapter 1 for a more complete discussion about what constitutes a healthy diet. It goes without saying

that a teacher should not smoke or use drugs (other than prescription medication) or misuse alcohol.

6. *Training in basic anatomy and the effects of Yoga techniques.* A teacher must be able to vary the techniques according to each student's ability and know how to advise students with common medical conditions such as hypertension, arthritis, and back problems. I also believe that a teacher should be able to recognize when a student needs professional psychological counseling.

7. *Ability to separate Yoga from religion.* Yoga is not an offshoot of Hinduism, as is commonly believed. The connection with Hinduism is a misconception based on the fact that Yoga developed in India and is reinforced by the many books about Yoga that have been written by people with a Hindu background who interpreted the principles of Yoga according to their personal belief systems. I have seen many poor-quality instructors take on the trappings and robes of Hinduism or some other religion to give themselves an authority through packaging rather

than through the authenticity of their own Yoga practice. Because there is so much misrepresentation of Yoga, and because we as Americans have no cultural background in self-development techniques, we are extremely vulnerable to such idealistic packaging and therefore are often misled by such poor leaders.

Yoga predates Hinduism—as well as all known religious practices—and its techniques have been used throughout the world. Yoga is a system of nonreligious, transcultural techniques that can develop greater self-knowledge and awareness. Unlike a religion, Yoga does not require adherence to certain creeds or beliefs, nor does it require obeisance to any particular prophet or god. Yoga is not ritualistic, nor is it occult. The texts of Yoga are not scriptures but rather handbooks or guidelines of how to use the techniques safely and what kinds of experiences might be possible. Everyone has a right to his or her personal religious beliefs, but a teacher must never impose his or her personal beliefs on students in a Yoga class.

A Last Word

Once I was in deep depression over the thought that one day Rama would die and leave me alone. When I expressed my sadness, he said to me, "Don't you know I am always with you? All you have to do is think of me, and I am there."

His words have sustained me many times over the years, as I have confronted the losses we all experience over a lifetime: people die or leave, expectations are shattered, hopes and dreams dissolve. Although loss still hurts, I have finally realized the truth of Rama's words: I cannot really lose anything. In the final analysis in real Yoga practice, the ultimate state is the knowledge that nothing can be lost and nothing gained; a state where there is no regret for losing anything and no desire for gaining anything.
Between these two poles is a vast silence where time changes and a deep happiness begins.

I never forget what Rama said to me many times: "Yoga makes the rough road smooth."

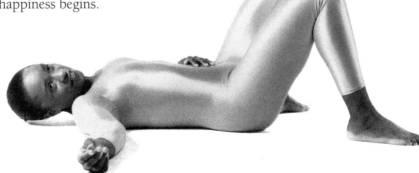

147

Appendix A:
A List of Asans with Sanskrit Names and Benefits

Alternate Big Sit-Up. *Padangusthasan* Variation. Strengthens transverse abdominal muscles, lower back, and shoulders; limbers and strengthens hip joints.

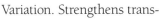

Alternate Seated Sun Pose. *Janu Sirasan*. Strengthens abdominal viscera and diaphragm; improves digestion; tones sympathetic nervous system; strengthens and stretches legs and spine; may help relieve impotence.

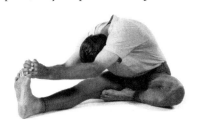

Alternate Triangle. *Trikona Hasthasan*. Localizes and stretches ligaments and nerves in the legs, back, and neck; improves circulation in entire pelvic region; reduces body fat in waist; stimulates intestines and kidneys; improves circulation in face and eyes.

Archer Pose.
Improves concentration and balance; strengthens willpower; increases mental clarity; strengthens muscles and joints in the feet, ankles, legs, and hips; helps repair damage caused by addiction.

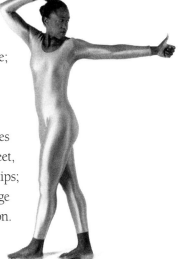

Arm and Leg Balance. Strengthens hip joints; improves balance; promotes correct posture; strengthens shoulders and upper back.

Baby Pose. *Virasan* Variation. Relieves stiffness in knees, hips, and ankles; improves digestion; improves functioning of reproductive system; limbers lower back; makes the mind bright and perceptive; gives clear, bright eyes and good complexion; gives energy to tolerate pain.

Big Sit-Up. *Padangusthasan.* Strengthens abdominal viscera and all abdominal and thigh muscles; improves balance and concentration; strengthens legs; improves digestion; strengthens eyesight.

Boat Pose. *Poorva Navasan.* Strengthens all back muscles and entire spinal column; stimulates digestion and functioning of all internal organs.

Bow Pose. *Dhanurasan.* Improves functioning of digestive system; strengthens and limbers back muscles and spinal column; increases vitality; develops heroism, courage, and endurance; improves concentration.

Bow Variation. *Dhanurasan* Variation. Strengthens vertebrae, back muscles, hips, thighs, and shoulders; improves posture, balance, and memory.

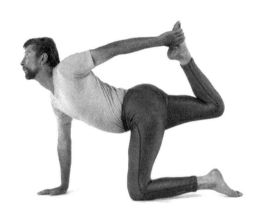

Camel Pose. *Ustrasan.* Limbers entire spine and pelvis; improves respiration; improves circulation in spinal column; stretches and strengthens upper and lower thighs and knees.

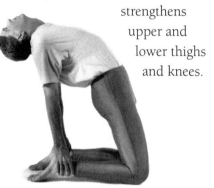

Candle Pose. *Sarvangasan* Variation. Tones endocrine system; removes fatigue; makes the mind bright and clear; enhances functioning of all vital organs; may improve reproductive function; improves eyesight; relieves tension in the heart and lungs; improves digestive function; brings independence and self-control; improves balance and concentration.

Cat Breath. Improves the action of intestines, heart, lungs, and liver; purifies blood; helps in management of hypertension; limbers spinal column; relieves tension in lower back; improves respiration.

Cat Variation. Same as above, plus: breaks up tense breath patterns; strengthens upper back, hip joints, and shoulders; limbers lower spine.

Cobra Pose. *Bhujangasan.* Improves functioning of intestines; increases body heat; strengthens back muscles and limbers spinal column; increases overall body strength; strengthens eyesight.

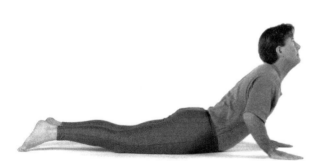

Cobra V-Raise. *Svanasan.* Strengthens legs, upper back, shoulders, and intercostal muscles; limbers and strengthens chest, neck, abdomen, and groin; improves functioning of internal organs; reduces body fat.

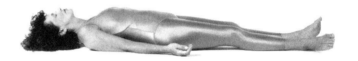

Corpse Pose. *Shavasan.* Removes fatigue; induces evenness of mind; reduces stress on nerves; makes inner organs function freely.

Crow Pose. *Kakasan.* Strengthens hands, wrists, arms, and shoulders; improves balance; relieves tension in heart and arteries.

Dancer Pose. *Natarajasan.* Strengthens lower back and lumbar vertebrae; stretches and strengthens hips and thighs; improves balance, poise, and concentration; removes phlegm and opens nasal passages; improves memory; relieves sluggishness and depression.

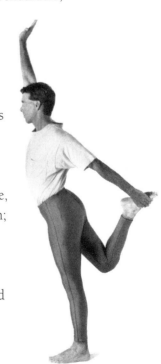

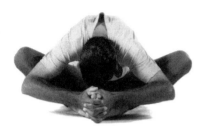

Diamond Pose.
Shiva Shaktiasan.
Tones and strengthens entire nervous system; strengthens and elongates sciatic nerve; improves digestion; strengthens and limbers hip joints; limbers lower back.

Eagle Pose.
Garudasan.
Strengthens legs and ankles; relieves stiffness in shoulders; prevents cramps in calf muscles; improves concentration and memory; makes one enterprising and swift.

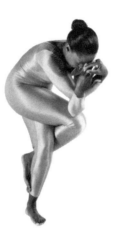

Easy Bridge. *Setau Bandhasan.*
Improves functioning of thyroid and parathyroid and entire endocrine system; eases back pain and fatigue; increases circulation to head and face, improving complexion and eyesight; may help in management of hypertension; helps relieve bedsores.

Fish Pose. *Matsyasan.* Fully expands chest for improved breathing and circulation; improves flexibility in neck and lower back; helps remove cal-

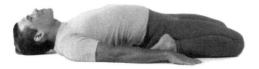

cium deposits from spinal column; helps relieve illnesses of throat; improves functioning of thyroid; strengthens eyesight; tones facial and throat muscles.

Full Bend. *Paschimottanasan*
Preparation. Tones and stretches nervous and muscular systems from the heels to the back of the head; improves circulation and respiration; strengthens rib cage, lungs, and heart muscles; helps to heal sciatic problems and varicose veins.

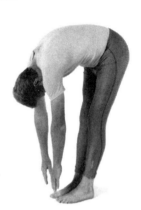

Hero Pose. *Virasan.* Elongates spinal nerves, spinal cord, and muscles of spinal column; stretches lower back; stretches and strengthens hips, knees, and ankles; elongates sciatic nerve and thigh muscles; gives courage.

Hero Compression.
Marichyasan.
Improves respiration and oxygenation of the blood; limbers hip, knee, and ankle joints; strengthens back and shoulder muscles.

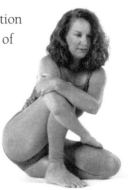

Locust Pose. *Salabasan.* Strengthens all back muscles and entire spinal column; improves digestion and functioning of vital organs; increases physical strength; reduces pain in sacral and lumbar regions; improves function of urinary system.

Lotus Pose. *Padmasan.* Keeps the back erect and the mind attentive and alert; relieves stiffness in the hips, knees, and ankles; brings all desired results and inclines the mind toward spiritual experience.

Lunge Series. *Hanumanasan* and Variations. Stretches and strengthens abductor muscles and hip joints; improves circulation to pelvis; improves reproductive function; elongates nerves and muscles in the legs.

One-Legged Sage Pose. *Ekapada Galavasan.* Strengthens arms and wrists; strengthens and limbers hip joints; improves balance and coordination; strengthens concentration and willpower.

Peacock Pose. *Mayurasan.* Tones abdominal region and improves circulation to all internal organs, especially liver, spleen, and intestines;

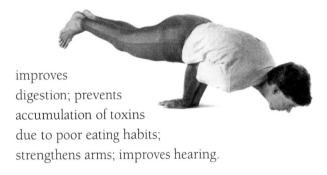

improves digestion; prevents accumulation of toxins due to poor eating habits; strengthens arms; improves hearing.

Pigeon Pose. *Rajakopotasan.* Stretches, strengthens, and tones spinal column and nerves, especially cervical and sacral vertebrae; strengthens and limbers hip joints and groin muscles; stimulates metabolic and reproductive glands and organs; increases vitality; may relieve impotence; strengthens and stretches rib cage and chest.

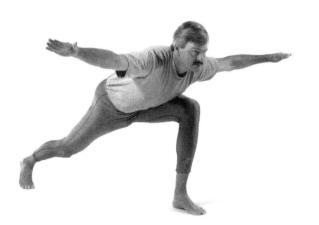

Plank Poses. *Vasisthasan.* Strengthens wrist, arm, shoulder, and neck muscles; improves circulation to entire body; strengthens back muscles and legs.

Plow Breath. *Halasan* Variation. Relieves tension in breath and midsection; strengthens abdominal, lower back, and leg muscles; stimulates function of internal organs.

Seated Sun Pose. *Paschimottanasan.* Strengthens abdominal viscera and diaphragm; improves digestive function; tones sympathetic nervous system; strengthens and stretches legs and spine; may help relieve impotence.

Shoulder Stand. *Sarvangasan.* Tones endocrine system; removes fatigue; makes the mind bright and clear; enhances functioning of all vital organs; may improve reproductive function; improves eyesight; relieves tension in the heart and lungs; improves digestive function; brings independence and self-control.

Side Crow Pose. *Parva Kakasan.* Strengthens arms, shoulders, wrists, and hands; improves functioning of the heart, lungs, stomach, and intestines; tones the sinus cavities in the nasal passages; improves balance; makes the spine elastic and strong.

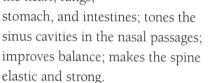

Side Stretch. Stretches transverse abdominal and intercostal muscles; limbers vertebrae; relieves tension in upper back and shoulders.

Side Triangle. *Uttihita Trikonasan.* Tones muscles of the legs and hips; stretches and develops the intercostal muscles; helps relieve backaches; strengthens back and neck.

Spine Twist. *Ardha Matsyendrasan.* Relieves chronic constipation; helps relieve urinary and prostate difficulties; strengthens rib cage and chest muscles; improves digestion; tones spinal nerves from base of spine to eyes; limbers hips and shoulders.

Standing Knee Squeeze. *Pavana Muktasan* Variation. Improves concentration and balance; relieves gas, constipation, and heartburn; improves circulation; reduces body fat in abdomen and thighs.

Standing Sun Pose. *Padahasthasan.* Stimulates functioning of all internal organs; improves circulation; strengthens and relieves tension on heart and lungs; limbers and strengthens muscles and nerves in back of legs and spine; increases strength.

T Pose. *Virbhadrasan.* Improves balance and concentration; strengthens

back and leg muscles; tones abdominal muscles and organs; increases mental poise.

"Telephone" Pose. *Ekapadasirasan.* Gives a perfect figure; limbers and stretches hip joints.

Tortoise Stretch. *Kurmasan.* Tones the spine; soothes the nerves of the brain; increases energy; develops

equanimity; renders the mind unswerving.

Tree Pose. *Vriksasan.* Strengthens legs; improves concentration and balance; improves respiration.

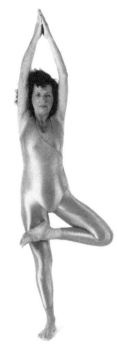

Triangle Poses. *Prasarita Padottanasan.* Limbers and strengthens hamstrings and abductor muscles; improves circulation and functioning of the internal organs; brings fresh blood to head, rejuvenating brain cells.

Twisting Triangle. *Parivritta Trikonasan.* Increases flexibility and circulation in lower spine and pelvis; strengthens hip joints; invigorates abdominal viscera and diaphragm; strengthens chest and neck; helps relieve depression.

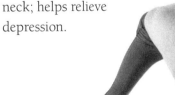

Warrior Pose. *Bhairavasan.*
Improves concentration and balance;
increases circulation throughout
body; strengthens leg muscles,
knees, and ankles; limbers shoulder
joints; improves posture; opens the
nerve centers in the spine.

Warrior Pose Variation. *Urdhva
Prasarita Ekapadasan.* Removes body
fat from waist, hips, and legs;
improves concentration and balance.

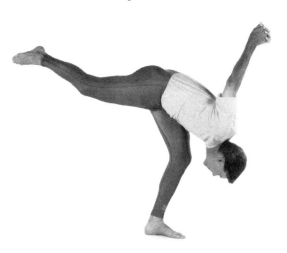

Wheel. *Chakrasan.* Tones the muscular, nervous, and circulatory systems;
increases
blood flow to
spine;
increases
energy to the
nerve centers
in the spine;
strengthens
nervous sys-
tem; helps to eliminate
toxins; improves strength and
willpower.

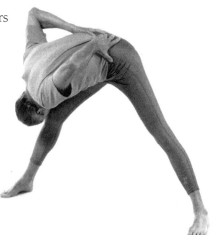

Windmill. Limbers
and strengthens
lower spine, hip
joints, and mus-
cles of upper
thigh; strengthens
lungs and breath-
ing muscles.

Appendix B:
Further Reading

You can extend your understanding of Yoga techniques and philosophy by studying any of the books listed below as well as other books and tapes by the American Yoga Association (see Appendix C). The following is by no means a complete list, but these are books that I believe will be most helpful to advancing students of Yoga. The best books to read are books that you enjoy reading; study should be a delight, not drudgery. Don't worry if you don't understand everything you read; my teacher Rama used to tell me to read anyway—even books written in other languages such as German or the original Sanskrit. He said that the information would affect my knowl-

edge of Yoga on levels other than my conscious awareness, and would be available when I needed it. I believed him then, and ever since, I have noticed that occasionally a thought or explanation will appear in my mind as if from nowhere, and I realize that the result of all those years of patient study is a treasure trove of knowledge lying in my unconscious mind like a gift that is being slowly unwrapped.

The *Bhagavad Gita*. Often called "the Yogi's handbook," this is eighteen chapters from a very long, ancient Indian epic called *The Mahabharata*. The *Bhagavad Gita* is available in many different translations, some with commentary. I suggest that you try to find a copy that is the least corrupted with the translator's religious interpretations.

Campbell, Joseph. *The Masks of God*, 4 volumes. Penguin (1968). A comprehensive study of world mythology incorporating art, religion, sociology, psychology, and history.

Campbell, Joseph. *The Hero with a Thousand Faces*. Princeton University Press (1968). A focused survey of the universal myth of the hero cycle as told in cultures around the world.

Danielou, Alain. *Yoga: Mastering the Secrets of Matter and the Universe*. Inner Traditions (1991). A clear explanation of the classical techniques of Yoga and some of the various kinds of Yoga.

Eliade, Mircea. *Yoga, Immortality and Freedom*. Princeton University Press (1969). An extensive discussion of the Yoga Sutras of Patanjali, including the aim of Yoga, the techniques and philosophies, the qualities of a student, and so on.

Rieker, Hans-Ulrich, Trans. *The Yoga of Light (Hatha Yoga Pradipika)*. Dawn Horse Press (1971). A translation of the classic text on Hatha Yoga.

Siva Samhita and *Gheranda Samhita*. These two ancient texts on Hatha Yoga are published only in India, as far as I know.

Woodruffe, Sir John. *Garland of Letters: Studies in the Mantra-Shastra. Discussions on Mantra Yoga—The Science of Sound*. Auromere (1969).

Zimmer, Heinrich. *Philosophies of India*. Princeton University Press (1951). A study of the major philosophical movements in India, including Yoga, Tantra, and Buddhism, among others.

Appendix C: Resources from the American Yoga Association

Further information on Yoga is available from the American Yoga Association. If you would like to write to us or obtain a free catalog, call or write:

American Yoga Association
513 South Orange Avenue
Sarasota, FL 34236-7501
Telephone (941) 954-3411 /
(800) 226-5859
Fax: (941) 364-9153
E-mail: Yogamerica@aol.com
Web site: *http://users.aol.com/
amyogaassn/aya.home/html*

We also offer classes in the Cleveland, Ohio, area. Information and schedules of local classes may be obtained by calling the toll-free number above.

Books

The American Yoga Association Beginner's Manual. Complete instructions for more than ninety Yoga exercises and breathing techniques; three ten-week curriculum outlines, and chapters on nutrition, philosophy, stress management, pregnancy, and more.

20-Minute Yoga Workouts: The Perfect Program for the Busy Person. Brief routines that anyone can fit into the busiest schedule. Includes chapters on women's issues, toning and shaping, the "20-minute challenge," and workouts to do when you're away from home.

The American Yoga Association Wellness Book. A basic routine to maintain health and well-being, plus chapters on how Yoga can specifically help with arthritis, heart disease, back pain, PMS, menopause, weight management, insomnia, headaches, and eight other health conditions.

Easy Does It Yoga. For those with physical limitations, this book includes instruction in specially adapted Yoga exercises that can be done in a chair or in bed, plus breathing techniques and meditation.

The Easy Does It Yoga Trainer's Guide. A complete manual for instruction in teaching the *Easy Does It Yoga* program to adults with physical limitations due to age, convalescence, substance abuse, injury, or obesity. Excellent for health professionals, activities directors, physical therapists, home health aides, and others who work with the elderly or in rehabilitative services.

Meditation. A collection of excerpts from Alice Christensen's lectures and classes on the subject of meditation, including a section of questions and answers from students.

Reflections of Love. A collection of excerpts from Alice Christensen's lectures and classes on the subject of love.

The Light of Yoga. A chronicle of the unusual circumstances that catapulted Alice Christensen into Yoga practice in the early 1950s, including the teachers and experiences that shaped her first years of study.

The Joy of Celibacy. This booklet examines how the unconscious is influenced by the sexual sell of modern advertising and suggests a five-minute celibacy break to help build awareness and self-knowledge.

Conversations with Swami Lakshmanjoo, Volume I: Aspects of Kashmir Shaivism. Edited transcripts of Alice Christensen's interviews with Swami Lakshmanjoo, who talks about his childhood and early years in Yoga, plus some basic concepts in the philosophy of Kashmir Shaivism.

Conversations with Swami Lakshmanjoo, Volume II: The Yamas and Niyamas of Patanjali. Edited transcripts of Alice Christensen's dialogues with Swami Lakshmanjoo about these essential ethical guidelines in Yoga.

Audiotapes

Complete Relaxation and Meditation with Alice Christensen. A two-tape audiocassette program that features three guided meditation sessions of varying lengths, including instruction in a seated posture, plus a discussion of meditation experiences.

The "I Love You" Meditation Technique. This technique begins with the experience of a more conscious connection with the breath through love. It then extends this feeling throughout the body and mind in relaxation and meditation. This tape teaches you the beauty of loving yourself and it removes unseen fear.

Videotapes

Basic Yoga. A complete introduction to Yoga that includes exercise, breathing, and relaxation and meditation techniques. Provides detailed instruction in all the techniques including variations for more or less flexibility, plus a special limbering routine and back-strengthening exercises. Features a thirty-minute practice session in a Yoga class setting for a convenient daily routine.

Conversations with Swami Lakshmanjoo. A set of three videotapes in which Alice Christensen introduces Swami Lakshmanjoo and talks with him about his background, the philosophy of Kashmir Shaivism, and other topics in Yoga.

(Some material corresponds to Volume I of the book *Aspects of Kashmir Shaivism* described above.)

The "I Love You" Meditation Technique. (See description under audiotapes.)

The Yamas and Niyamas: A Videotape Study Program. A complete set of twenty-five videotapes of Alice Christensen's comprehensive lectures on the ethical guidelines that form the cornerstone of Yoga philosophy and practice. Includes a study guide.

The Hero in Yoga: A Videotape Study Program. A series of twenty-four videotaped lectures by Alice Christensen on Joseph Campbell's landmark text *The Hero with a Thousand Faces,* showing how the adventure of the hero, represented in mythologies all over the globe, parallels the Yoga student's search for self-actualization. Includes a study guide.

Index

About the American Yoga Association

The American Yoga Association teaches a comprehensive and balanced program of Yoga that includes Hatha Yoga exercises and breathing techniques as well as meditation. Rather than stressing physical culture for its own sake, our core curriculum acknowledges the deeper possibilities of Yoga by teaching meditation and encouraging the inner-directed awareness that eventually leads to greater self-knowledge, producing a powerful individual. This reliance on individual experience and feeling is a central theme in the science of Yoga, and it underlies the philosophical system of Kashmir Shaivism, which supports our line of teaching.

Our goal is to offer the highest quality Yoga instruction possible. There are two American Yoga Association Centers in the United States.

About the Author

Alice Christensen stands out as a Yoga teacher with the rare ability to make the often complex ideas and techniques of Yoga accessible to our Western outlook and lifestyle. She established the American Yoga Association in 1968, then the first and only nonprofit organization in the United States dedicated to education in Yoga.

She has consistently presented Yoga in a clear, classical manner for over forty years. She presents Yoga without dogma or prescription, as a potent avenue for individual inquiry. She has designed programs of Yoga that can be used to enhance any lifestyle. Whether the goal is to maintain health or to explore the nature of the self, her programs can be used to achieve a wide range of goals.